W9-BVE-965

Nutrition for Nursing
Review Module Edition 5.0

CONTRIBUTORS

Sheryl Sommer, PhD, RN, CNE
VP Nursing Education & Strategy

Janean Johnson, MSN, RN
Nursing Education Strategist

Karin Roberts, PhD, MSN, RN, CNE
Nursing Education Coordinator

Sharon R. Redding, EdD, RN, CNE
Nursing Education Specialist and Content Project Coordinator

Lois Churchill, MN, RN
Nursing Education Specialist

Brenda Ball, MEd, BSN, RN
Nursing Education Specialist

Norma Jean Henry, MSN/Ed, RN
Nursing Education Specialist

Peggy Leehy, MSN, RN
Nursing Education Specialist

Mendy G. McMichael, DNP, MSN, RN
Nursing Education Specialist

EDITORIAL AND PUBLISHING

Derek Prater
Spring Lenox
Michelle Renner
Mandy Tallmadge
Kelly Von Lunen

CONSULTANTS

Justina Higgins, RN, MSN, PLNC, HCE, CHC
Honey C. Holman, MSN, RN

Intellectual Property Notice

Important Notice to the Reader

User's Guide

Welcome to the Assessment Technologies Institute® Nutrition for Nursing Review Module Edition 5.0. The mission of ATI's Content Mastery Series® review modules is to provide user-friendly compendiums of nursing knowledge that will:

- Help you locate important information quickly.
- Assist in your learning efforts.
- Provide exercises for applying your nursing knowledge.
- Facilitate your entry into the nursing profession as a newly licensed RN.

Organization

This review module is organized into units covering principles of nutrition, clinical nutrition, and alterations in nutrition. Chapters within these units conform to one of three organizing principles for presenting the content:

- Nursing concepts
- Procedures
- Disorders

Nursing concepts chapters begin with an overview describing the central concept and its relevance to nursing. Subordinate themes are covered in outline form to demonstrate relationships and present the information in a clear, succinct manner.

Procedures chapters include an overview describing the procedure(s) covered in the chapter. These chapters will provide you with nursing knowledge relevant to each procedure, including indications, interpretation of findings, nursing actions, and complications.

Disorders chapters include an overview describing the disorder(s) and the relation to nutrition. These chapters cover assessment and nutritional guidelines and nursing interventions, including preventive and therapeutic nutrition.

Application Exercises

Questions are provided at the end of each chapter so you can practice applying your knowledge. The Application Exercises include NCLEX-style questions, such as multiple-choice and multiple-select items, and questions that ask you to apply your knowledge in other formats, such as by using an ATI Active Learning Template. After the Application Exercises, an answer key is provided, along with rationales for the answers.

NCLEX® Connections

To prepare for the NCLEX-RN, it is important for you to understand how the content in this review module is connected to the NCLEX-RN test plan. You can find information on the detailed test plan at the National Council of State Boards of Nursing's Web site: https://www.ncsbn.org/. When reviewing content in this review module, regularly ask yourself, "How does this content fit into the test plan, and what types of questions related to this content should I expect?"

To help you in this process, we've included NCLEX Connections at the beginning of each unit and with each question in the Application Exercises Answer Keys. The NCLEX Connections at the beginning of each unit will point out areas of the detailed test plan that relate to the content within that unit. The NCLEX Connections attached to the Application Exercises Answer Keys will demonstrate how each exercise fits within the detailed content outline.

These NCLEX Connections will help you understand how the detailed content outline is organized, starting with major client needs categories and subcategories and followed by related content areas and tasks. The major client needs categories are:

- Safe and Effective Care Environment
  - Management of Care
  - Safety and Infection Control
- Health Promotion and Maintenance
- Psychosocial Integrity
- Physiological Integrity
  - Basic Care and Comfort
  - Pharmacological and Parenteral Therapies
  - Reduction of Risk Potential
  - Physiological Adaptation

An NCLEX Connection might, for example, alert you that content within a unit is related to:

- Basic Care and Comfort
  - Nutrition and Oral Hydration
    - Manage the client who has an alteration in nutritional intake.

QSEN Competencies

As you use the review modules, you will note the integration of the Quality and Safety Education for Nurses (QSEN) competencies throughout the chapters. These competencies are integral components of the curriculum of many nursing programs in the United States and prepare you to provide safe, high-quality care as a newly licensed RN. Icons appear to draw your attention to the six QSEN competencies which include:

- Safety: The minimization of risk factors that could cause injury or harm while promoting quality care and maintaining a secure environment for clients, self, and others.
- Patient-Centered Care: The provision of caring and compassionate, culturally sensitive care that addresses clients' physiological, psychological, sociological, spiritual, and cultural needs, preferences, and values.

- Evidence Based Practice: The use of current knowledge from research and other credible sources, on which to base clinical judgment and client care.
- Informatics: The use of information technology as a communication and information-gathering tool that supports clinical decision making and scientifically based nursing practice.
- Quality Improvement: Care related and organizational processes that involve the development and implementation of a plan to improve health care services and better meet clients' needs.
- Teamwork and Collaboration: The delivery of client care in partnership with multidisciplinary members of the health care team, to achieve continuity of care and positive client outcomes.

Icons

Icons are used throughout the review module to draw your attention to particular areas. Keep an eye out for these icons:

 This icon is used for NCLEX connections.

 This icon is used for content related to safety and is a QSEN competency. When you see this icon, take note of safety concerns or steps that nurses can take to ensure client safety and a safe environment.

 This icon is a QSEN competency which indicates the important of a holistic approach to providing care.

 This icon, a QSEN competency, points out the integration of research into clinical practice.

 This icon is a QSEN competency and highlights the use of information technology to support nursing practice.

 This icon is used to focus on the QSEN competency of integrating planning processes to meet clients' needs.

 This icon highlights the QSEN competency of care delivery using an interprofessional approach.

 This icon indicates that a media supplement, such as a graphic, an animation, or a video, is available. If you have an electronic copy of the review module, this icon will appear alongside clickable links to media supplements. If you have a hardcopy version of the review module, visit www.atitesting.com for details on how to access these features.

Feedback

ATI welcomes feedback regarding this review module. Please provide comments to: comments@atitesting.com.

TABLE OF CONTENTS

UNIT 1   Principles of Nutrition

CHAPTERS

› Sources of Nutrition
› Ingestion, Digestion, Absorption, and Metabolism
› Nutrition Assessment
› Guidelines for Healthy Eating
› Food Safety
› Cultural, Ethnic, and Religious Influences
› Nutrition Across the Lifespan

NCLEX® CONNECTIONS

When reviewing the chapters in this unit, keep in mind the relevant sections of the NCLEX® outline, in particular:

Client Needs: Health Promotion and Maintenance

› Relevant topics/tasks include:
  » Aging Process
    › Provide care and education that meets the special needs of the preschool client ages 1 year to 3 years.
  » Ante/Intra/Postpartum and Newborn Care
    › Provide prenatal care and education.
  » Health and Wellness
    › Identify the client's health-oriented behaviors.

Client Needs: Basic Care and Comfort

› Relevant topics/tasks include:
  » Nutrition and Oral Hydration
    › Calculate the client's intake and output.
    › Initiate calorie counts for clients.
    › Apply knowledge of mathematics to client nutrition.

chapter 1

Overview

- Nutrients absorbed in the diet determine, to a large degree, the health of the body. Deficiencies or excesses can contribute to a poor state of health. Essential nutrients are those that the body cannot manufacture, and the absence of essential nutrients can cause deficiency diseases.

- Components of nutritive sources are:
  - Carbohydrates and fiber
  - Protein
  - Lipids (fats)
  - Vitamins
  - Minerals and electrolytes
  - Water

- Carbohydrates, fats, and proteins are all energy-yielding nutrients.

- Dietary Reference Intakes (DRIs), are developed by the Institute of Medicine's Food and Nutrition Board, and are the most commonly used source on nutrient allowances for healthy individuals. Formerly known as the Recommended Dietary Allowances (RDAs), the DRIs are comprised of four reference values: RDAs, Estimated Average Requirements (EARs), Adequate Intakes (AIs), and Tolerable Upper Intake Levels (ULs).

CARBOHYDRATES AND FIBER

- All carbohydrates are organic compounds composed of carbon, hydrogen, and oxygen (CHO). The main function of carbohydrates is to provide energy for the body.

  - The average minimum amount of carbohydrates needed to fuel the brain is 130 g/day. Median carbohydrate intake is 200 to 330 g/day among men and 180 to 230 g/day among women. The acceptable macronutrient distribution range for carbohydrates is 45% to 65% of calories.

  - Carbohydrates provide energy for cellular work, and help to regulate protein and fat metabolism. They are essential for normal cardiac and central nervous system (CNS) functioning.

  - Carbohydrates are classified according to the number of saccharide units making up their structure.
    - Monosaccharides are simple carbohydrates (glucose, fructose).
    - Disaccharides are simple carbohydrates (sucrose, lactose).
    - Polysaccharides are complex carbohydrates (starch, fiber, glycogen).

  - As complex carbohydrates are ingested and broken down, they are easily absorbed in the intestine and into the bloodstream where they are stored in the liver and muscles for energy needs.

  - The body absorbs 80% to 95% of carbohydrates. Absorption occurs mainly in the small intestine using pancreatic and intestinal enzymes.

  - Glycogen is the stored carbohydrate energy source found in the liver and muscles. It is a vital source of backup energy.

- ○ Carbohydrates provide 4 cal/g of energy.
- ○ Fiber is categorized as a carbohydrate, but it does not yield energy for the body.
  - ▪ Dietary fiber is the substance in plant foods that is indigestible. Types are pectin, gum, cellulose, and mucilage.
  - ▪ Fiber is important for proper bowel elimination. It adds bulk to the feces and stimulates peristalsis to ease elimination.
  - ▪ Studies show fiber helps to lower cholesterol and lessen the incidence of intestinal cancers.

TYPES OF CARBOHYDRATES		
Type	Example (Sources)	Function
› Monosaccharides	› Glucose (corn syrup), fructose (fruits), galactose (milk sugar broken down)	› Basic energy for cells
› Disaccharides	› Sucrose (table sugar, molasses), lactose (milk sugar), maltose (sweeteners)	› Energy, aids calcium and phosphorus absorption (lactose)
› Polysaccharides	› Starches (grains, legumes, root vegetables), fiber (indigestible plant parts)	› Energy storage (starches), digestive aid (fiber)

PROTEINS

- • Proteins are provided by plant and animal sources. They are formed by linking amino acids in various combinations for specific use by the body.
  - ○ There are three types of proteins: complete, incomplete, and complementary. Each is obtained from the diet in various ways.
    - ▪ Complete proteins, generally from animal sources, contain all of the essential amino acids (there are nine essential amino acids).
    - ▪ Incomplete proteins, generally from plants (grains, nuts, legumes, vegetables, fruits), do not contain all of the essential amino acids.
    - ▪ Complementary proteins are those food sources that, when eaten together, provide all the essential amino acids.
  - ○ Proteins have many metabolic functions (tissue-building and maintenance, balance of nitrogen and water, backup energy, support of metabolic processes [nitrogen balance, transportation of nutrients, other vital substances], support of the immune system).
  - ○ Three main factors influence the body's requirement for protein:
    - ▪ Tissue growth needs.
    - ▪ Quality of the dietary protein.
    - ▪ Added needs due to illness.
  - ○ The recommended dietary requirement of protein for adults is 10% of intake, or 46 g/day for women and 56 g/day for men.
  - ○ Undernutrition may lead to protein malnourishment, which can lead to kwashiorkor or marasmus. These serious disorders are caused by a lack of protein ingestion, or the metabolism resulting in a cachectic (wasting) state.
  - ○ Protein provides 4 cal/g of energy.

LIPIDS

- The chemical group of fats is called lipids, and they are available from many sources (dark meat, poultry skin, dairy foods, and added oils [margarine, butter, shortening, oils, lard]).
  - Fat is an essential nutrient for the body. It serves as a concentrated form of energy for the body (second to carbohydrates) and supplies important tissue needs (hormone production, structural material for cell walls, protective padding for vital organs, insulation to maintain body temperature, covering for nerve fibers, aid in the absorption of fat-soluble vitamins).
  - Fats are divided into the following categories: triglycerides, phospholipids, sterols, saturated fats, unsaturated fats, polyunsaturated fats, and essential fatty acids.
    - Triglycerides (the chemical name for fats) are the primary form of fat in food. They combine with glycerol to supply energy to the body, allow fat-soluble vitamin transport, and form adipose tissue that protects the body.
    - Phospholipids are derived from triglycerides. They are important to cell membrane structure.
    - Cholesterol belongs to the chemical substance group called sterols. It is necessary for cell membrane stability and the production of certain hormones and bile salts for digestion. If cholesterol is consumed in excess, it can build up in the tissues causing congestion and increasing the risk for cardiovascular disease.
    - Saturated fats are of animal origin. Unsaturated fats are usually from plant sources and help reduce health risks (notable exceptions are coconut and palm oil).
    - Essential fatty acids, made from broken down fats, must be supplied by the diet. Essential fatty acids, including omega-3 and omega-6, are used to support blood clotting, blood pressure, inflammatory responses, and many other metabolic processes.
    - Linoleic acid is an important essential fatty acid and is found primarily in polyunsaturated vegetable oils.
  - Generally, no more than 20% to 35% of total calories should come from fat (10% or less from saturated fat sources).
    - A diet high in fat is linked to cardiovascular disease, hypertension, and diabetes mellitus.
    - The exception is for children under 2 years of age, who need a higher amount of fat to form brain tissue.
  - Conversely, a diet with less than 10% fat cannot supply adequate amounts of essential fatty acids and results in a cachectic (wasting) state.
  - The majority of lipid metabolism occurs after fat reaches the small intestine, where the gallbladder secretes concentrated bile and acts as an emulsifier to break fat into smaller particles. At the same time, the pancreas secretes pancreatic lipase, which breaks down fat. The small intestine secretes an enzyme for further breakdown. The muscles, liver, and adipose tissue cause the release of fatty acids, and the liver produces lipoproteins to carry lipids.
    - Very-low-density lipoproteins (VLDL) carry triglycerides to the tissues.
    - Low-density lipoproteins (LDL) carry cholesterol to the tissues.
    - High-density lipoproteins (HDL) remove excess cholesterol from the tissues. HDL is considered "good" cholesterol.
  - Lipids provide 9 cal/g of energy and are the densest form of stored energy.

VITAMINS

- Vitamins are organic substances required for many enzymatic reactions. The main function of vitamins is to be a catalyst for metabolic functions and chemical reactions.
  - There are 13 essential vitamins, each having a specialized function.
  - The two classes of vitamins are:
    - Water-soluble – Vitamins C and B-complex
    - Fat-soluble – Vitamins A, D, E, and K
  - Vitamins yield no usable energy for the body.
- Water-Soluble Vitamins
  - Vitamin C (ascorbic acid) aids in tissue building and metabolic reactions (wound and fracture healing, collagen formation, adrenaline production, iron absorption, conversion of folic acid, cellular adhesion).
    - Vitamin C is found in citrus fruits (oranges, lemons), tomatoes, peppers, green leafy vegetables, and strawberries.
    - Stress and illness increase the need for vitamin C.
    - Severe deficiency causes scurvy, a hemorrhagic disease with diffuse tissue bleeding, painful limbs/joints, weak bones, and swollen gums/loose teeth.
  - B-complex vitamins have many functions in cell metabolism. Each one has a varied duty. Many partner with other B vitamins for metabolic reactions. Most affect energy, metabolism, and neurological function. Sources for B vitamins almost always include green leafy vegetables and unprocessed or enriched grains.
    - Thiamin (B_1) is necessary for proper digestion, peristalsis, and providing energy to the smooth muscles, glands, the CNS, and blood vessels.
      - Deficiency results in beriberi, gastrointestinal findings, and cardiovascular problems.
      - Food sources are widespread in almost all plant and animal tissues, especially meats, grains, and legumes.
    - Riboflavin (B_2) is required for growth and tissue healing.
      - Deficiency results in cheilosis (manifestations include scales and cracks on lips and mouth), smooth/swollen red tongue, and dermatitis particularly in skin folds.
      - Dietary sources include milk, meats, and green leafy vegetables.
    - Niacin (B_3) aids in the metabolism of fats, glucose, and alcohol.
      - Deficiency causes pellagra (manifestations include sun-sensitive skin lesions, and gastrointestinal and neurological findings).
      - Sources include beef liver, nuts, legumes, whole grain and enriched breads and cereals.
    - Pantothenic acid (B_5) is involved in biological reactions (energy production, catabolism, and synthesis of fatty acids, phospholipids, cholesterol, steroid hormones, the neurotransmitter acetylcholine).
      - Deficiency results in anemia and CNS changes. However, a deficiency is unlikely due to the diverse availability in foods.
      - Rich sources include organ meats (liver, kidney), egg yolk, avocados, cashew nuts and peanuts, brown rice, soy, lentils, broccoli, and milk.

- Pyridoxine (B_6) is needed for cellular function and synthesis of hemoglobin, neurotransmitters, and niacin.
  - Deficiency causes anemia and CNS disturbances.
  - High intake of supplements may cause sensory neuropathy.
  - Widespread food sources include organ meats and grains.
- Biotin serves as a coenzyme used in fatty acid synthesis, amino acid metabolism, and the formation of glucose.
  - Deficiency is rare, but results in neurological findings (depression, fatigue) and rashes on the skin, especially the face ("biotin deficient face").
  - Widespread food sources include eggs, milk, and dark green vegetables.
- Folate (folic acid is the synthetic form) is required for hemoglobin and amino acid synthesis, cellular reproduction, and prevention of neural tube defects in utero.
  - Deficiency causes megaloblastic anemia, CNS disturbances, and fetal neural tube defects (spina bifida and anencephaly). It is important that all women of child-bearing age get an adequate amount of folate due to neural tube formation occurring early in gestation, often before a woman knows she is pregnant.
  - Folate occurs naturally in a variety of foods including liver, dark-green leafy vegetables, citrus fruits, whole-grain products, and legumes.
- Cobalamin (B_{12}) is necessary for the production of red blood cells.
  - Deficiency causes pernicious anemia and is seen mostly in strict vegetarians (B_{12} is found solely in foods of animal origin), and those with the absence of intrinsic factor needed for the absorption of B_{12}.
  - Sources include beef liver, shellfish, and fortified grains.

WATER-SOLUBLE VITAMINS AT A GLANCE		
MAJOR ACTIONS	MAJOR SOURCES	DEFICIENCY
Vitamin C (ascorbic acid)		
› Antioxidant, tissue building, iron absorption	› Citrus fruits and juices, vegetables	› Scurvy, decreased iron absorption, bleeding gums
Thiamin (B_1)		
› Muscle energy, GI support, CV support	› Meats, grains, legumes	› Beriberi, altered digestion, CNS and CV problems
Riboflavin (B_2)		
› Growth, energy, tissue healing	› Milk, meats, green leafy vegetables	› Skin eruptions, cracked lips, red swollen tongue
Niacin (B_3)		
› Energy and protein metabolism/ cellular metabolism	› Liver, nuts, legumes	› Pellagra, skin lesions, GI and CNS findings, dementia
Pantothenic acid (B_5)		
› Fatty acid metabolism, cell synthesis, heme production	› Organ meats, egg yolk, avocados, broccoli	› Anemia, CNS changes

| WATER-SOLUBLE VITAMINS AT A GLANCE | | |
MAJOR ACTIONS	MAJOR SOURCES	DEFICIENCY
Pyridoxine (B$_6$)		
› Cellular function, heme and neurotransmitter synthesis	› Organ meats, grains	› Anemia, CNS hyper-irritability, dermatitis
Folate		
› Synthesis of amino acids and hemoglobin, lower neural tube defect in fetus	› Liver, green leafy vegetables, grains, legumes	› Megaloblastic anemia, CNS disturbance
Cobalamin (B$_{12}$)		
› Hemoglobin synthesis, fatty acid metabolism	› Organ meats, clams, oysters, grains	› Pernicious anemia, GI findings, poor muscle coordination

- Fat-Soluble Vitamins
  - All fat-soluble vitamins have the possibility for toxicity due to their ability to be stored in the body for long periods of time.
  - Absorption of fat-soluble vitamins is dependent on the body's ability to absorb dietary fat.
    - Fat digestion can be interrupted by any number of conditions, particularly those that affect the secretion of fat-converting enzymes, and conditions of the small intestine. Clients who have cystic fibrosis, celiac disease, Crohn's disease, or intestinal bypasses are at risk for deficiencies.
  - Clients who have liver disease should be careful not to take more than the daily recommendations of fat-soluble vitamins, as levels can build up.
  - Vitamin A (retinol, beta-carotene) contributes to vision health, tissue strength and growth, and embryonic development.
    - Care should be taken when administered to pregnant clients as some forms have teratogenic effects on the fetus.
    - Deficiency results in vision changes, xerophthalmia (dryness and thickening of the conjunctiva), and changes in epithelial cells (especially in the mouth and vaginal mucosa).
    - Food sources include fish liver oils, egg yolks, butter, cream, and dark yellow/orange fruits and vegetables (carrots, yams, apricots, squash, cantaloupe).
  - Vitamin D (calciferol) assists in the utilization of calcium and phosphorus, and aids in skin repair. It can be used preventively for immune function.
    - Sunlight enables the body to synthesize vitamin D.
    - Deficiency results in bone demineralization, and extreme deficiency results in rickets. Clients on glucocorticoid therapy may require additional amounts. Excess consumption may cause hypercalcemia.
    - Food sources include fortified milk, cod liver oil, and eggs.
    - Low vitamin D levels may increase the risk for chronic diseases, such as multiple sclerosis, type I diabetes mellitus, hypertension, and certain cancers.

- Vitamin E (tocopherol) is an antioxidant that helps to preserve muscles and red blood cells, and maintains the myelin sheath that insulates nerve cells.
  - Deficiency results in hemolytic anemia and affects the nerve fibers that influence walking and vision.
  - Food sources include vegetable oils and certain nuts.
- Vitamin K (menaquinone, phylloquinone) assists in blood clotting and bone maintenance.
  - Deficiency results in increased bleeding time.
  - Used as an antidote for excess anticoagulants (warfarin [Coumadin]).
  - Vitamin K is found in some oils, liver, and green leafy vegetables (spinach, broccoli, cabbage). The typical American diet provides adequate amounts.

FAT-SOLUBLE VITAMINS AT A GLANCE		
MAJOR ACTIONS	MAJOR SOURCES	DEFICIENCY
Vitamin A		
› Normal vision, tissue strength, growth and tissue healing	› Orange/yellow colored foods, liver, dairy	› Reduced night vision, dry/thick eyes, mucosa changes
Vitamin D		
› Maintain serum calcium and phosphorus, aid in bone development	› Fish, fortified dairy products, sunlight	› Low serum calcium, fragile bones, rickets
Vitamin E		
› Protects cells from oxidation	› Vegetable oils, grains, nuts, dark green vegetables	› Hemolytic anemia, CNS changes
Vitamin K		
› Normal blood clotting (prothrombin production), aids in bone metabolism	› Green leafy vegetables, eggs, liver	› Increased bleeding times

MINERALS AND ELECTROLYTES

- Minerals are available in an abundance of food sources and are used at every cellular level for metabolic exchanges.
  - Minerals are divided into major and trace.
    - Major minerals occur in larger amounts in the body.
    - Trace elements, also called micronutrients, are required by the body in amounts of less than 100 mg/day.
  - The seven major minerals are calcium, phosphorus, sodium, potassium, magnesium, chloride, and sulfur.
  - The 10 trace elements are iron, iodine, zinc, copper, manganese, chromium, cobalt, selenium, molybdenum, and fluoride.
  - Electrolytes are electrically charged minerals that cause physiological reactions that maintain homeostasis. The most commonly monitored electrolytes are sodium, potassium, chloride, calcium, and magnesium. They affect many disease processes.

MAJOR MINERALS AT A GLANCE

SODIUM (Na)

Major Actions	› Maintains fluid volume, allows muscle contractions, cardiovascular support
Major Sources	› Table salt, added salts, processed foods, butter
Findings of Deficiency	› Muscle cramping, cardiac changes
Findings of Excess	› Fluid retention, hypertension, CVA
Nursing Implications	› Monitor ECG, edema, and blood pressure.

POTASSIUM (K)

Major Actions	› Maintains fluid volume inside/outside cells, muscle action, blood pressure, cardiovascular support
Major Sources	› Oranges, dried fruits, tomatoes, avocados, dried peas, meats, broccoli, bananas
Findings of Deficiency	› Dysrhythmias, muscle cramps, confusion
Findings of Excess	› Dysrhythmias (caused by supplements, potassium-sparing diuretics, ACE inhibitors, inadequate kidney function, diabetes)
Nursing Implications	› Monitor ECG and muscle tone. PO tabs irritate the GI system. Give with meals.

CHLORIDE (Cl)

Major Actions	› Bonds to other minerals (especially sodium) to facilitate cellular actions and reactions, fluid balance
Major Sources	› Table salt
Findings of Deficiency	› Rare
Findings of Excess	› In concert with sodium, results in high blood pressure
Nursing Implications	› Monitor sodium levels.

CALCIUM (Ca)

Major Actions	› Bones/teeth, cardiovascular support, blood clotting, nerve transmission
Major Sources	› Dairy, broccoli, kale, grains, egg yolks
Findings of Deficiency	› Osteoporosis, tetany, Chvostek's and Trousseau's signs, ECG changes
Findings of Excess	› Constipation, kidney stones
Nursing Implications	› Monitor ECG and muscle tone. Give PO tabs with vitamin D.

MAGNESIUM (Mg)

Major Actions	› Bone nourishment, catalyst for many enzyme reactions, nerve/muscle function, CV support
Major Sources	› Green leafy vegetables, nuts, grains, meat, milk
Findings of Deficiency	› Weakness, dysrhythmias, tetany, seizure, reduced blood clotting, eclampsia
Findings of Excess	› Diarrhea, kidney stones, decreased muscle control, CV changes
Nursing Implications	› Incompatible with some antibiotics. Give PO, 2 hr apart.

MAJOR MINERALS AT A GLANCE	
PHOSPHORUS (P)	
Major Actions	› Energy transfer of RNA/DNA, acid-base balance, bone and teeth formation
Major Sources	› Dairy, peas, soft drinks, meat, eggs, some grains
Findings of Deficiency	› Calcium level changes, muscle weakness
Findings of Excess	› Skeletal porosity, decreased calcium levels, must stay in balance with calcium
Nursing Implications	› Evaluate the use of antacids (note type) and the use of alcohol.
SULFUR (S)	
Major Actions	› A component of vitamin structure, by-product of protein metabolism
Major Sources	› Dried fruits (dates, raisins, apples), meats, red and white wines
Findings of Deficiency	› Only seen in severe protein malnourishment, found in all protein-containing foods
Findings of Excess	› Toxicity has a very low risk
Nursing Implications	› Sulfur levels are not usually monitored.

- ○ Select Trace Minerals
  - Iodine is used for synthesis of thyroxine, the thyroid hormone that helps regulate metabolism. Iodine is taken up by the thyroid. When iodine is lacking, the thyroid gland enlarges, creating a goiter.
    - □ Grown food sources vary widely and are dependent on the iodine content of the soil in which they were grown.
    - □ Seafood provides a good amount of iodine. Table salt in the U.S. is fortified with iodine, so deficiencies are not as prevalent.
    - □ The RDA is 100 to 150 mcg for adults.
  - Iron is responsible for hemoglobin formation/function, cellular oxidation of glucose, antibody production, and collagen synthesis.
    - □ The body "scavenges" unused iron from dying red blood cells and stores it for later use.
    - □ Iron supplements may cause constipation, nausea, vomiting, diarrhea, and teeth discoloration (liquid form). They should be taken with food to avert gastrointestinal symptoms, and nurses should encourage fresh fruits, vegetables, and a high-fiber diet.
    - □ Supplements that are unneeded can become toxic.
    - □ Intramuscular injections are caustic to tissues and must be administered by Z-track method.
    - □ Food sources include organ meats, egg yolks, whole grains, and green leafy vegetables.
    - □ Vitamin C increases the absorption of iron.
    - □ The greatest need for iron is the newborn who is not breastfed, and for females during the menstruating years.
  - Fluoride forms a bond with calcium and thus accumulates in calcified body tissue (bones and teeth). Water with added fluoride protects against dental cavities. Nurses should instruct clients who prefer to drink bottled water that they may need fluoride treatments from their dentist.

WATER

- Water is the most basic of nutrients. The body can maintain itself for several days or weeks on its food stores of energy, but it cannot survive without water/hydration for more than a few days. Water makes up the largest portion of our total body weight and is crucial for all fluid and cellular functions.

  ○ Fluid balance is essential for optimum health and bodily function.

  ○ The balance of fluid is a dynamic process regulated by the release of hormones.

  ○ To maintain a balance between intake and output, intake should approximate output. The minimum daily total fluid output in healthy adults is 1,500 mL. Therefore, the minimum daily amount of water needed is 1,500 mL.

  ○ Under normal conditions, recommended adult fluid intake is 3 to 4 L/day for men and 2 to 3 L/day for women. It is recommended that half be from water.

  ○ Additional hydration may be required for athletes, persons with fever/illness (vomiting, diarrhea), and those in hot climate conditions.

  ○ Young children and older adults dehydrate more rapidly.

  ○ Clients who cannot hold down fluid or must withhold fluids in preparation for a procedure may be hydrated with intravenous fluids.

  ○ Water leaves the body via the kidneys, skin, lungs, and feces. The greatest elimination is through the kidneys. Other loss factors to be considered include bleeding, vomiting, and rapid respirations. Persistent vomiting can quickly dehydrate a person.

  ○ A balanced input/output ratio is almost 1:1. Nurses should consider the health status and individual needs of the client.

  ○ Assessment for proper hydration should include skin turgor, mental status, orthostatic blood pressures, urine output and concentration, and moistness of mucous membranes.

   ○ Thirst is a late sign of the need for hydration, especially in older adults.

  ○ Some individuals may have an aversion to drinking water, and should be encouraged to explore other options (fresh fruits, fruit juices, flavored gelatin, frozen treats, soups).

  ○ Caffeinated drinks have a diuretic effect and should not be substituted for other drinks.

APPLICATION EXERCISES

1. A nurse is educating a client who is taking iron supplements about foods which aid in iron absorption. Which of the following food choices indicates an understanding of the teaching?

    A. Baked potato

    B. Orange juice

    C. Milk

    D. Green beans

2. A nurse is discussing foods that are high in vitamin D with a client who is unable to be out in the sunlight. Which of the following should be included in the teaching?

    A. Tacos and rice

    B. Hamburgers and fried potatoes

    C. Ham and Brussels sprouts

    D. Eggs and fortified milk

3. A nurse is caring for a client who is prescribed warfarin (Coumadin). Which of the following food choices should the nurse advise the client to limit?

    A. Orange juice

    B. Broccoli

    C. Ice cream

    D. Chicken

4. A nurse is conducting a nutritional class on minerals and electrolytes. Which of the following food sources should be included when discussing magnesium?

    A. Nuts

    B. Tomatoes

    C. Canned soup

    D. Yogurt

5. A nurse is discussing health problems associated with nutrient deficiencies. Which of the following conditions is associated with a deficiency of vitamin C?

    A. Dysrhythmias

    B. Scurvy

    C. Pernicious anemia

    D. Megaloblastic anemia

6. A school nurse is conducting a nutritional class for a group of athletes. Use the ATI Active Learning Template: Basic Concept to complete this item to describe three types of protein and three main factors influencing the body's requirement for protein.

APPLICATION EXERCISES KEY

1.   A. INCORRECT: A baked potato does not aid in the absorption of iron.

   B. **CORRECT:** Vitamin C aids in the absorption of iron, and orange juice is a good source of vitamin C.

   C. INCORRECT: Milk does not aid in the absorption of iron.

   D. INCORRECT: Green beans do not aid in the absorption of iron.

   Ⓝ NCLEX® Connection: Basic Care and Comfort, Nutrition and Oral Hydration

2.   A. INCORRECT: Tacos and rice do not provide vitamin D.

   B. INCORRECT: Hamburgers and fried potatoes do not provide vitamin D.

   C. INCORRECT: Ham and Brussels sprouts do not provide vitamin D.

   D. **CORRECT:** Sunlight helps synthesize vitamin D, so clients need egg yolks and fortified milk, which are both good sources of vitamin D.

   Ⓝ NCLEX® Connection: Basic Care and Comfort, Nutrition and Oral Hydration

3.   A. INCORRECT: Orange juice does not effect coagulation.

   B. **CORRECT:** Broccoli is a green leafy vegetable and is a good source of vitamin K. The client should avoid excess vitamin K because it has a negative response to warfarin effects.

   C. INCORRECT: Ice cream does not effect coagulation.

   D. INCORRECT: Chicken does not effect coagulation.

   Ⓝ NCLEX® Connection: Basic Care and Comfort, Nutrition and Oral Hydration

4.   A. **CORRECT:** Nuts are a good source of magnesium and should be included in the teaching.

   B. INCORRECT: Tomatoes are a good source of potassium.

   C. INCORRECT: Canned soup contains sodium.

   D. INCORRECT: Yogurt is a good source of calcium.

   Ⓝ NCLEX® Connection: Physiological Adaptations, Fluid and Electrolyte Imbalances

5. A. INCORRECT: Dysrhythmias are associated with a potassium deficiency.

    B. **CORRECT:** Scurvy is associated with a vitamin C deficiency.

    C. INCORRECT: Pernicious anemia is associated a deficiency of vitamin B_{12}.

    D. INCORRECT: Megaloblastic anemia is associated with a deficiency of folate.

    Ⓝ NCLEX® Connection: Physiological Adaptations, Fluid and Electrolyte Imbalances

6. *Using the ATI Active Learning Template: Basic Concept*
    - Types of Protein
      - Complete proteins, generally from animal sources, contain all of the essential amino acids (there are nine essential amino acids).
      - Incomplete proteins, generally from plants (grains, nuts, legumes, vegetables, fruits), do not contain all of the essential amino acids.
      - Complementary proteins are those food sources that, when eaten together, provide all the essential amino acids.
    - Main Factors Influencing the Body's Requirement for Protein
      - Tissue growth needs
      - Quality of the dietary protein
      - Added needs due to illness

    Ⓝ NCLEX® Connection: Health Promotion and Maintenance, Health Promotion/Disease Prevention

chapter 2

Overview

- Ingestion is the process of consuming food by the mouth, and moving it through the digestive system.
- Digestion is a systemic process that includes the breakdown and absorption of nutrients.
- Absorption occurs as components of nutrients pass through the digestive system into the bloodstream and lymphatic system.
  - Medication absorption can be affected by food intake. It is important for nurses to be aware of food and medication absorption.
  - Nurses should assess liver and kidney functioning to determine adequacy prior to medication administration.
- Metabolism is the sum of all chemical processes that occur on a cellular level to maintain homeostasis. Nutrients from food must enter a cell in order for metabolism to occur.
  - Metabolism is comprised of two processes: catabolism, the breaking down of substances with the resultant release of energy, and anabolism, the use of energy to build or repair substances.
  - Energy nutrients are metabolized to provide carbon dioxide, water, heat, and adenosine triphosphate (ATP).
  - Excess energy nutrients are stored; glucose is converted to glycogen and stored in the liver and muscle tissue; surplus glucose is converted to fat; glycerol and fatty acids are reassembled into triglycerides and stored in adipose tissue; and amino acids make body proteins. The liver removes excess amino acids and uses the residue to form glucose or store it as fat.
  - Body cells first use available ATP for growth and repair, then use glycogen and stored fat.

Metabolic Rate

- Metabolic rate refers to the speed at which food energy is burned. Basal metabolic rate (BMR), also called resting energy expenditure (REE), refers to the amount of energy used when the body is at rest.
  - BMR/REE also are interchangeable with basal energy expenditure (BEE).
- BMR is primarily affected by lean body mass and hormones. Body surface area, age, and gender are minor factors as they relate to body mass index (BMI).

FACTORS AFFECTING BMR	INCREASE BMR	DECREASE BMR
Lean, muscular body build	✓	
Short, overweight body build		✓
Starvation/malnutrition		✓
Exposure to extreme cold	✓	

FACTORS AFFECTING BMR	INCREASE BMR	DECREASE BMR
Prolonged stress	✓	
Rapid growth periods (infancy, puberty)	✓	
Pregnancy	✓	
Lactation	✓	
Over 60 years of age		✓
Physical conditioning	✓	

- In general, men have a higher metabolic rate than women because of their higher amount of body muscle and decreased amount of fat.
- Thyroid function tests may be used as an indirect measure of BMR.
- Acute stress causes an increase in metabolism, blood glucose levels, and protein catabolism.
  - The major nutritional concern during acute stress is protein deficiency as stress hormones break down protein at a very rapid rate.
  - Protein deficiency increases the risk of complications from severe trauma or critical illness (skin breakdown, delayed wound healing, infections, organ failure, ulcers, impaired drug tolerance).
  - Protein requirements may be increased to 2.0 g/kg of body weight depending on the client's age and prior nutritional status.
  - Inadequate protein intake prevents the body from adapting to physiologic stress.
- Alcohol is more quickly metabolized and absorbed than nutrients. Alcohol metabolism changes liver cells and reduces the liver's ability to metabolize fat. Alcoholics suffer from protein-energy malnutrition, generally consuming about 75% of energy requirements, resulting in low to normal albumin levels.
- Any catabolic illness (surgery, extensive burns) increases the body's requirement for calories to meet the demands of an increased BMR.
- Disease and sepsis also increase metabolic demands and can lead to starvation/death.

CONDITIONS THAT AFFECT METABOLIC RATE		
CONDITION	INCREASES METABOLISM	DECREASES METABOLISM
Fever	✓	
Involuntary muscle tremors, as in shivering or Parkinson's	✓	
Hypothyroidism		✓
Hyperthyroidism	✓	
Cancer	✓	
Cardiac failure	✓	
Some anemias	✓	
Hypertension	✓	
Chronic obstructive pulmonary disease	✓	

CONDITIONS THAT AFFECT METABOLIC RATE		
CONDITION	INCREASES METABOLISM	DECREASES METABOLISM
Burns	✓	
Surgery/wound healing	✓	
HIV/AIDS	✓	

MEDICATIONS THAT AFFECT THE BODY'S RATE OF METABOLISM		
MEDICATION	INCREASES BMR	DECREASES BMR
Somatropin (Genotropin)	✓	
Prednisone (Deltasone)	✓	
Hydrocortisone (Cortef)	✓	
Epinephrine hydrochloride	✓	
Levothyroxine sodium (Synthroid)	✓	
Glucagon	✓	
Ephedrine sulfate	✓	
Amitriptyline (Elavil)		✓

Nitrogen Balance

- Nitrogen balance refers to the difference between the daily intake and excretion of nitrogen. It is also an indicator of tissue integrity. A healthy adult experiencing a stable weight is in nitrogen equilibrium, also known as neutral nitrogen balance.

- Positive nitrogen balance indicates that the intake of nitrogen exceeds excretion. Specifically, the body builds more tissue than it breaks down. This normally occurs during periods of growth: infancy, childhood, adolescence, pregnancy, and lactation.

- Negative nitrogen balance indicates that the excretion of nitrogen exceeds intake. The individual is receiving insufficient protein, and the body is breaking down more tissue than it is building, as seen in illness, trauma, immobility, and malnutrition.

- Clinical signs of negative nitrogen balance are not immediately evident. Decreased muscle tissue, impaired organ function, and increased susceptibility to infection are late signs.

Nursing Assessments/Data Collection

- Weight and history of recent weight patterns
- Medical history for diseases that affect metabolism and nitrogen balance
- Extent of traumatic injuries, as appropriate
- Fluid and electrolyte status
- Abnormal laboratory values: albumin, transferrin, glucose, and creatinine

- Clinical signs of malnutrition: pitting edema, hair loss, and wasted appearance
- Medication side effects that can affect nutrition
- Usual 24 hr diet intake
- Use of nutritional supplements, herbal supplements, vitamins, and minerals
- Use of alcohol, caffeine, and nicotine

Nursing Interventions

- Provide adequate calories and high quality protein. Strategies to increase protein and caloric content include:
  - Add skim milk powder to milk (double-strength milk).
  - Substitute whole milk for water in recipes.
  - Add cheese, peanut butter, chopped hard-cooked eggs, or yogurt to foods.
  - Dip meats in eggs or milk and coat with bread crumbs before cooking.
  - Nuts and beans are significant sources of protein. These are good alternatives for a dairy allergy or lactose intolerance.
- Monitor food intake.
- Monitor fluid intake and output.

- Use patient-centered approach to address disease-specific problems with ingestion, digestion, or medication regime.
- Collaborate with nutritionist.

APPLICATION EXERCISES

1. A nurse is caring for a client who has hypothyroidism. Which of the following clinical findings are associated with this disorder?

    A. Decreased metabolic demand

    B. Weight loss

    C. Increased heart rate

    D. Diarrhea

2. A nurse is reviewing prescribed medications for a newly admitted client. Which of the following medications decreases the body's rate of metabolism?

    A. Prednisone (Deltasone)

    B. Levothyroxine (Synthroid)

    C. Amitriptyline (Elavil)

    D. Somatropin (Genotropin)

3. A charge nurse is conducting a nutritional class for a group of newly licensed nurses regarding basal metabolic rate (BMR). The charge nurse should inform the class that which of the following increases BMR? (Select all that apply.)

_____   A. Lactation

_____   B. Prolonged stress

_____   C. Malnutrition

_____   D. Puberty

_____   E. Exposure to extreme cold

4. A nurse is caring for a client who is immobilized because of bilateral femur and tibia fractures. Which of the following are clinical signs of negative nitrogen balance? (Select all that apply.)

_____   A. Decreased muscle tissue

_____   B. Impaired organ function

_____   C. Increased susceptibility to infection

_____   D. Increased metabolism

_____   E. Decreased protein catabolism

5. A nurse is conducting a nutritional program for a group of newly licensed nurses regarding ingestion, digestion, absorption, and metabolism. Use the ATI Active Learning Template: Basic Concept to complete this item by identifying three components of absorption.

APPLICATION EXERCISES KEY

1. A. **CORRECT:** Hypothyroidism causes a decreased metabolic demand.

    B. INCORRECT: Weight gain is a clinical finding associated with hypothyroidism.

    C. INCORRECT: Bradycardia a clinical finding associated with hypothyroidism.

    D. INCORRECT: Constipation is clinical finding associated with hypothyroidism.

    Ⓝ NCLEX® Connection: Health Promotion and Maintenance, Aging Process

2. A. INCORRECT: Prednisone is a glucocorticoid used for suppressing the immune system and inflammation. This medication increases the body's rate of metabolism.

    B. INCORRECT: Levothyroxine is used for the treatment of hypothyroidism and increases the body's rate of metabolism.

    C. **CORRECT:** Amitriptyline is tricyclic antidepressant used for treating depression and decreases the body's rate of metabolism.

    D. INCORRECT: Somatropin is used as a growth hormone and increases the body's rate of metabolism.

    Ⓝ NCLEX® Connection: Physiological Adaptations, Illness Management

3. A. **CORRECT:** Lactation increases BMR and should be included in the teaching.

    B. **CORRECT:** Prolonged stress increases BMR and should be included in the teaching.

    C. INCORRECT: Malnutrition decreases BMR and should not be included in the teaching.

    D. **CORRECT:** Puberty increases BMR and should be included in the teaching.

    E. **CORRECT:** Exposure to extreme cold increases BMR because the body uses more energy to regulate the body temperature.

    Ⓝ NCLEX® Connection: Health Promotion and Maintenance, Aging Process

4. A. **CORRECT:** Decreased muscle tissue is a clinical sign of negative nitrogen balance.

    B. **CORRECT:** Impaired organ function is a clinical sign of negative nitrogen balance.

    C. **CORRECT:** Increased susceptibility to infection is a clinical sign of negative nitrogen balance.

    D. **CORRECT:** Increased metabolism is a clinical sign of negative nitrogen balance.

    E. INCORRECT: Protein catabolism increases during acute stress.

    (N) NCLEX® Connection: Physiological Adaptations, Illness Management

5. *Using the ATI Active Learning Template: Basic Concept*
    - Three Components of Absorption
        - Absorption occurs as components of nutrients pass through the digestive system into the bloodstream and lymphatic system.
        - Medication absorption can be affected by food intake. It is important for nurses to be aware of food and medication absorption.
        - Nurses should assess liver and kidney functioning to determine adequacy prior to medication administration.

    (N) NCLEX® Connection: Health Promotion and Maintenance, Aging Process

UNIT 1   PRINCIPLES OF NUTRITION

CHAPTER 3   Nutrition Assessment

Overview

- Nurses play a key role in assessing the nutritional needs of clients.
  - ○ Nurses monitor and intervene with clients requiring acute and chronic nutritional care.
  - ○ The family's nutritional habits must be considered and incorporated into a client's individual plan of care.
  - ○ Nurses should take an active role in surveying and teaching community groups regarding nutrition.

- A collaborative, interprofessional approach provides the best outcomes for the client.
  - ○ Physical assessment data is collected by providers and nurses.
  - ○ Comprehensive nutritional assessments are completed by registered dieticians.
  - ○ Nurses monitor and evaluate interventions provided to clients.
- A client's physical appearance can be deceiving.
  - ○ A client with a healthy weight and appearance can be malnourished.
  - ○ Cultural, social, and physical norms must be part of a client's assessment.
- Even with adequate client education, personal preferences can be an overriding factor to successful nutritional balance.

Diet History

- A diet history is an assessment of usual foods, fluids, and supplements. Components include:
  - ○ Time, type, and amount of food eaten for breakfast, lunch, dinner, and snacks.
  - ○ Time, type, and amount of fluids consumed throughout the day, including water, health drinks, coffee/tea, carbonated beverages, and beverages with caffeine.
  - ○ Type, amount, and frequency of "special foods" (celebration foods, movie foods).
  - ○ Typical preparation of foods and fluids (coffee with sugar, fried foods).
  - ○ Number of meals eaten away from home (at work or school).
  - ○ Type of normal diet (ovo-lacto vegetarian, 2 g sodium/low-fat diet).
  - ○ Foods avoided due to allergy or preference.
  - ○ Frequency and dose/amount of medications or nutritional supplements taken daily.
  - ○ Satisfaction with diet over a specified time frame (last 3 months, 1 year).

Assessment Tools to Determine Nutritional Status

- A physical assessment is performed by the provider or nurse to identify indicators of inadequate nutrition. However, clinical findings may be caused by other processes, diseases, or conditions. Manifestations include:
  - Hair that is dry or brittle, or skin that has dry patches.
  - Poor wound healing or sores.
  - Lack of subcutaneous fat or muscle wasting.
  - Abnormal cardiovascular measurements (heart rate and rhythm, blood pressure).
  - General weakness or impaired coordination.
- Anthropometric Tools
  - Weight
    - Weigh at the same time of day wearing similar clothing to ensure accurate weight readings.
    - Daily fluctuations generally are indicative of water weight changes.
    - Percentage weight change calculation (weight change over a specified time):

      $$\frac{\text{usual weight} - \text{present weight}}{\text{usual weight}} \times 100$$

      - 1% to 2% in 1 week indicates a significant weight loss.
      - 7.5% in 3 months indicates a significant weight loss.
    - "Ideal" body weight based on height (plus or minus 10% depending on frame size).
      - For males, 48 kg (106 lb) for the first 152 cm (5 ft) of height, and 2.7 kg (6 lb) for each additional 2.5 cm (1 in).
      - For females, 45 kg (100 lb) for the first 152 cm (5 ft) of height, and 2.3 kg (5 lb) for each additional 2.5 cm (1 in).
  - Height
    - Young children and infants should be measured lying on a firm, flat surface.
  - Body Mass Index (BMI)
    - Normal/healthy weight is indicated by a BMI of 18.5 to 24.9.
    - Overweight is defined as an increased body weight in relation to height. It is indicated by a BMI of 25 to 29.9.
    - Obesity is an excess amount of body fat. It indicated by a BMI greater than or equal to 30.
    - BMI = weight (kg) ÷ height (m^2)
- Clinical Values
  - Fluid intake and output (I&O)
  - Adults – 2,000 to 3,000 mL (2 to 3 L) per day
  - Total average output – 2,300 to 2,600 mL/day

- ○ Protein levels commonly are measured by serum albumin levels. Many non-nutritional factors (injury or kidney disease), interfere with this measure for protein malnutrition.

- ○ Prealbumin (thyroxin-binding protein) is a more susceptible measure used to assess critically ill clients who are at a higher risk for malnutrition. This test reflects more acute changes rather than gradual changes. However, it is more expensive and often unavailable. This is not part of routine assessment.

CLINICAL LABORATORY TESTS	NORMAL	MODERATE DEPLETION
Albumin	3.5 to 5.0 g/dL	2.1 to 2.7 g/dL
Prealbumin	23 to 43 mg/dL	5 to 9 mg/dL

Risk Factors for Inadequate Nutrition

- Biophysical Factors
  - ○ Medical disease/conditions/treatment (hypertension, HIV/AIDS, surgery)
  - ○ Genetic predisposition (lactose intolerance, osteoporosis)
  - ○ Age
- Psychological Factors
  - ○ Mental illness (clinical depression)
  - ○ Excessive stress
  - ○ Negative self-concept
  - ○ Use of comfort foods
- Socioeconomic Factors
  - ○ Poverty
  - ○ Alcohol and drug use disorders
  - ○ Fad or "special" diets
  - ○ Food preferences: cultural, ethnic, or religious
- Impact of Risk Factors on Nutritional Status
  - ○ The following are examples of how risk factors can affect nutritional status.
    - A client is edematous and requires treatment with a diuretic and low-sodium diet. Diuretics can cause sodium and potassium imbalances. A low-sodium diet may be unappetizing and cause inadequate consumption. Salt substitutes in moderation may be used to add flavor.
    - Osteoporosis has many modifiable risk factors (calcium and vitamin D intake, inactive lifestyle, cigarette smoking, alcohol intake). Altering these risk factors can affect nutritional status in a positive manner.
    - Poor self-concept may cause a client to avoid needed foods and nutrients, or to overeat.

APPLICATION EXERCISES

1. A nurse in a nutritional clinic is calculating body mass index (BMI) for several clients. Which of the following BMI represents an overweight client?

    A. 24

    B. 30

    C. 27

    D. 32

2. A nurse is caring for a client on an orthopedic unit who sustained trauma in a motor-vehicle crash. Which of the following laboratory values indicates moderate protein deficiency?

    A. Serum albumin 3.5 g/dL

    B. Serum prealbumin 5 mg/dL

    C. Serum albumin 4.5 g/dL

    D. Serum prealbumin 10 mg/dL

3. A nurse is performing a nutritional assessment on a client. Which of the following clinical findings are suggestive of malnutrition? (Select all that apply.)

    _____ A. Poor wound healing

    _____ B. Dry hair

    _____ C. Blood pressure 130/80 mm Hg

    _____ D. Weak hand grips

    _____ E. Impaired coordination

4. A nurse is teaching a nutritional class to a group of women. Which of the following should the nurse include as risk factors for developing osteoporosis? (Select all that apply.)

    _____ A. Inactivity

    _____ B. Familiar history

    _____ C. Obesity

    _____ D. Hyperlipidemia

    _____ E. Cigarette smoking

5. A community health nurse is conducting a dietary assessment for a client. Use the ATI Active Learning Template: Basic Concept to complete this item to describe four components of a diet history.

APPLICATION EXERCISES KEY

1. A. INCORRECT: Normal/healthy weight is indicated by a BMI of 18.5 to 24.9.

    B. INCORRECT: Obesity is an excess amount of body fat indicated by a BMI greater than or equal to 30.

    C. **CORRECT:** Overweight is defined as an increased body weight in relation to height, indicated by a BMI of 25 to 29.9.

    D. INCORRECT: Obesity is an excess amount of body fat indicated by a BMI greater than or equal to 30.

    Ⓝ NCLEX® Connection: Basic Care and Comfort, Nutrition and Oral Hydration

2. A. INCORRECT: Serum albumin levels reflect slow changes in serum protein levels, not acute serum protein changes. A serum albumin of 3.5 g/dL or 4.5 g/dL is within the normal range.

    B. **CORRECT:** A serum prealbumin level of 5 mg/dL is indicative of a moderate depletion of protein. The serum prealbumin test, also known as thyroxin-binding protein, is the most sensitive to acute changes in protein nutrition.

    C. INCORRECT: Serum albumin levels reflect slow changes in serum protein levels, not acute serum protein changes. A serum albumin of 3.5 g/dl or 4.5 g/dL is within the normal range.

    D. INCORRECT: A serum prealbumin of 10 mg/dL is indicative of a mild depletion of protein.

    Ⓝ NCLEX® Connection: Reduction of Risk Potential, Laboratory Values

3. A. **CORRECT:** Poor wound healing describes changes reflective of malnutrition.

    B. **CORRECT:** Dry hair describes changes reflective of malnutrition.

    C. INCORRECT: A blood pressure value of 130/80 mm Hg is an expected cardiovascular finding and is not associated with malnutrition.

    D. **CORRECT:** Weak hand grips describe changes reflective of malnutrition.

    E. **CORRECT:** Impaired coordination describe changes reflective of malnutrition.

    Ⓝ NCLEX® Connection: Basic Care and Comfort, Nutrition and Oral Hydration

4. A. **CORRECT:** There is an increased risk for osteoporosis due to inactivity. Weight-bearing exercises should be discussed as primary prevention measures.

    B. **CORRECT:** Osteoporosis runs in families.

    C. INCORRECT: Weight loss can cause a decreased intake of dietary calcium and vitamin D, leading to the development of osteoporosis.

    D. INCORRECT: Hyperlipidemia is not a risk factor for the development of osteoporosis in women.

    E. **CORRECT:** Cigarette smoking may increase the incidence of osteoporosis.

    Ⓝ NCLEX® Connection: Health Promotion and Maintenance, Health Promotion/Disease Prevention

5. *Using the ATI Active Learning Template: Basic Concept*
    - A diet history is an assessment of usual foods, fluids, and supplements.
        ○ Time, type, and amount of food eaten for breakfast, lunch, dinner, and snacks.
        ○ Time, type, and amount of fluids consumed throughout the day including water, health drinks, coffee/tea, carbonated beverages, and beverages with caffeine.
        ○ Type, amount, and frequency of "special foods" (celebration foods, movie foods).
        ○ Typical preparation of foods and fluids (coffee with sugar, fried foods).
        ○ Number of meals eaten away from home (at work or school).
        ○ Type of normal diet (ovo-lacto vegetarian, 2 g sodium/low-fat diet).
        ○ Foods avoided due to allergy or preference.
        ○ Frequency and dose/amount of medications or nutritional supplements taken daily.
        ○ Satisfaction with diet over a specified time frame (last 3 months, year).

    Ⓝ NCLEX® Connection: Health Promotion and Maintenance, Health Screening

chapter 4

Overview

- Nutrition is vital to maintaining optimal health. Healthy food choices and controlling weight are important steps in promoting health and reducing risk factors for disease.

- Nurses should encourage favorable nutritional choices, and can serve as informational resources for clients regarding guidelines for healthy eating.

- Established guidelines for healthy eating that clients and nurses can refer to include the Dietary Guidelines for Americans and MyPlate, along with a number of condition- or system-specific guidelines.

- Vegetarian diets can meet all nutrients recommendations. It is essential to consume a variety and correct amount of foods to meet individual caloric needs.

The Dietary Guidelines for Americans

- The U.S. Department of Agriculture (USDA) and the U.S. Department of Health and Human Services (HHS) publish the Dietary Guidelines for Americans jointly every 5 years. It provides research-based advice concerning food intake and physical activity for healthy Americans over 2 years of age. The updates can be found at www.cnpp.usda.gov/DietaryGuidelines.htm or www.health.gov/dietaryguidelines.

- The Dietary Guidelines for Americans advocates healthy food selections: a variety of fiber-rich fruits and vegetables, whole grains, low-fat or fat-free milk and milk products, lean meats, poultry, fish, legumes, eggs, and nuts. Recommendations include "nutrient-dense" foods.

  - Balance energy intake with energy expenditure by selecting a wide variety of foods, and limiting saturated and transaturated fat, sugars, sodium, and alcohol.

  - Establish exercise routines to promote cardiovascular health, muscle strength and endurance, and psychological well-being.

  - Increase consumption of fiber-rich fruits and vegetables to a minimum of five servings per day in order to decrease risk factors for certain cancers. The vitamin and mineral content of these foods may decrease the risk of DNA damage and cancer.

  - Choose monounsaturated and polyunsaturated fats from fish, lean meats, nuts, and vegetable oils. Fat intake may average 30% of total caloric intake with less than 10% from saturated fats. Avoid synthetic/solid fats (oils preferred).

  - Limit sugar and starchy foods to decrease the occurrence of dental caries.

  - Consume less than 2,300 mg of salt per day (about 1 tsp) by limiting most canned and processed foods. Prepare foods without adding salt.

  - Drink alcohol in moderation: up to one drink per day for women and two per day for men. Certain medical conditions, medication therapies, and physical activities preclude the use of alcohol.

  - Follow food safety guidelines when preparing, cooking, and storing food. Avoid consumption of raw eggs and unpasteurized milk and juices.

MyPlate

- The USDA sponsors a Web site that promotes healthy food choices balanced with physical activity (www.choosemyplate.gov). The pyramid is based on the current USDA dietary guidelines, and is a tool to help individuals identify daily amounts of foods based on criteria (age, gender, activity level). The five food groups represented are grains, vegetables, fruit, dairy, and protein foods.

FOOD GROUP	RECOMMENDED SERVINGS (2,000-CALORIE DIET)	REPRESENTATIVE FOODS
Grains	6 oz	Whole-grain breads, cereals, rice, pasta One slice bread = 1 oz 1 cup cereal = 1 oz ½ cup cooked pasta = 1 oz
Vegetables	2 ½ cups (raw, cooked, or juice)	Broccoli, carrots, dry beans and peas, corn, potatoes, tomatoes
Fruits	2 cups	One small banana, orange ¼ cup dried apricots
Milk	3 cups (2 cups for children ages 2 to 8 years)	2% milk, yogurt, cheese
Protein foods	5 ½ oz	Beef, poultry, eggs, kidney beans, soy beans, fish, nuts and seeds, peanut butter One small chicken breast = 3 oz One egg = 1 oz ¼ cup dried cooked beans = 1 oz
Oils	6 tsp	Canola oil, corn oil, olive oil, nuts, olives, some fish

 View Image: MyPlate

- MyPlate can serve as a reminder to balance calorie intake with suitable activity.
  - Adults should engage in at least 2.5 hr each week of moderate level aerobic physical activity or 1.25 hr each week of vigorous level aerobic physical activity.
  - Children and adolescents should be physically active for 60 min/day.

Vegetarian Diets

- A vegetarian diet focuses on plants for food, including fruits, vegetables, dried beans and peas, grains, seeds, and nuts. There is no single type of vegetarian diet. Vegetarian eating patterns usually fall into the following groups:
  - The vegan diet excludes all meat and animal products.
  - The lacto vegetarian diet includes dairy products.
  - The lacto-ovo vegetarian diet includes dairy products and eggs.
- People who follow vegetarian diets can get all the nutrients they need, but they must be careful to eat a wide variety of foods to meet their nutritional needs. Nutrients vegetarians may need to focus on include protein, iron, calcium, zinc, and vitamin B_{12}.

Food Labels

- The Food and Drug Administration (FDA) requires certain information be included with packaged foods and beverages. The information is included on the Nutrition Facts label or food label, which is a boxed label found on foods and beverages. Food labels must include single serving size, number of servings in the package, percent of daily values, and the amount of each nutrient in one serving.
- Nutrients included on the food label:
  - Calories
  - Calories from fat
  - Total fat
  - Saturated fat
  - Trans fat
  - Cholesterol
  - Sodium
  - Total carbohydrates
  - Dietary fiber
  - Sugars
  - Protein
  - Vitamin A
  - Vitamin C
  - Calcium
  - Iron
- Clients should be taught to read food labels properly to ensure individual nutritional needs are met, and healthy choices are made.

 View Video: Understanding Food Labels

Strategies for Promotion of Specific Areas of Health

- Healthy hearts
  - ○ Limit saturated fat to 10% of calories and cholesterol to 300 mg/day.
  - ○ For individuals with elevated low density lipoproteins (LDL), the American Heart Association (AHA) recommends increasing monounsaturated fats and soluble fiber.
  - ○ The Dietary Approaches to Stop Hypertension (DASH) diet has been proven by research to significantly lower systolic and diastolic blood pressure.
- Healthy nervous systems
  - ○ Normal functioning of the nervous system depends on adequate levels of the B-complex vitamins, especially thiamin, niacin, and vitamins B_6 and B_{12}.
  - ○ Calcium and sodium are important regulators of nerve responses. Consuming the recommended servings from the grain and dairy food groups provides these nutrients.
- Healthy bones
  - ○ Consuming the recommended servings from the MyPlate's dairy group supplies the calcium, magnesium, and phosphorus necessary for bone formation, and vitamin D that aids in the absorption of calcium and phosphorus.
  - ○ Weight-bearing physical activity is essential to decrease the risk of osteoporosis.
- Good bowel function
  - ○ Normal bowel functioning depends on adequate fluid intake and 25 g/day of fiber for women, and 38 g/day for men.
  - ○ The minimum number of servings from MyPlate's fruit, vegetable, and grain food groups (specifically whole grains) provides the essential nutrients.
- Cancer prevention
  - ○ A well-balanced diet using MyPlate and a healthy weight are guidelines to prevent cancer.
  - ○ Increase high-fiber plant-based foods.
  - ○ Limit saturated and polyunsaturated fat, while emphasizing foods with monounsaturated fat or omega-3 fatty acids (nuts and fish).
  - ○ Limit sodium intake.
  - ○ Avoid excess alcohol intake.
  - ○ Include regular physical activity.

APPLICATION EXERCISES

1. A nurse is teaching a client measures for healthy bones. Which of the following statements by the client requires additional teaching?

    A. "I will eat foods high in calcium."

    B. "I will increase my fluid intake."

    C. "I should participate in weight bearing exercises."

    D. "I should get my vitamin D from the sunlight."

2. A nurse is conducting a nutritional class to a group of newly licensed nurses. Which of the following should be included in the teaching?

    A. Limit saturated fat to 10% of total caloric intake.

    B. Good bowel function requires 35 g/day of fiber for women.

    C. Limit cholesterol consumption to 400 mg/day.

    D. Normal functioning cardiac systems depends on B-complex vitamins.

3. A nurse is discussing essential nutrients for normal functioning of the nervous system. Which of the following should be included in the teaching? (Select all that apply.)

    _____ A. Calcium

    _____ B. Thiamin

    _____ C. Vitamin B_6

    _____ D. Sodium

    _____ E. Phosphorus

4. A school nurse is teaching a group of students how to read food labels. Which of the following should be included in the teaching? (Select all that apply.)

    _____ A. Total carbohydrates

    _____ B. Total fat

    _____ C. Calories

    _____ D. Magnesium

    _____ E. Dietary fiber

5. A community health nurse is conducting a nutritional class regarding cancer prevention strategies. Use the ATI Active Learning Template: Basic Concept to complete this item to describe four components recommended to prevent cancer.

APPLICATION EXERCISES KEY

1. A. INCORRECT: Calcium is necessary for healthy bone formation.

   B. **CORRECT:** Increasing fluid intact does not promote healthy bones. Additional client teaching is indicated.

   C. INCORRECT: Weight-bearing physical activity is essential to decrease the risk of osteoporosis.

   D. INCORRECT: Vitamin D is necessary for calcium absorption and health bone formation.

   Ⓝ NCLEX® Connection: Health Promotion and Maintenance, Health Promotion/Disease Prevention

2. A. **CORRECT:** Saturated fat should be limited to 10% of total caloric intake.

   B. INCORRECT: Good bowel function requires 25 g/day of fiber for women, and 38 g/day for men.

   C. INCORRECT: Cholesterol consumption should be limited to 300 mg/day.

   D. INCORRECT: Normal functioning nervous system depends on B-complex vitamins.

   Ⓝ NCLEX® Connection: Health Promotion and Maintenance, Health Promotion/Disease Prevention

3. A. **CORRECT:** Calcium is an important regulator of nerve responses.

   B. **CORRECT:** Normal functioning of the nervous system depends on adequate levels of the B-complex vitamins, especially thiamin, niacin, and vitamins B_6 and B_{12}.

   C. **CORRECT:** Normal functioning of the nervous system depends on adequate levels of the B-complex vitamins, especially thiamin, niacin, and vitamins B_6 and B_{12}.

   D. **CORRECT:** Sodium is an important regulator of nerve responses.

   E. INCORRECT: Phosphorus is not important for normal functioning of the nervous system.

   Ⓝ NCLEX® Connection: Health Promotion and Maintenance, Health Promotion/Disease Prevention

4. A. **CORRECT:** The Food and Drug Administration (FDA) requires certain information be included with packaged foods and beverages. Total carbohydrates are included on food labels.

    B. **CORRECT:** Food labels must include single serving size, number of servings in the package, percent of daily values, and the amount of each nutrient in one serving. Total total fat is included on food labels.

    C. **CORRECT:** Calories are included on food labels.

    D. INCORRECT: Magnesium is not included on food labels.

    E. **CORRECT:** Dietary fiber is included on food labels.

    Ⓝ NCLEX® Connection: Health Promotion and Maintenance, Aging Process

5. *Using the ATI Active Learning Template: Basic Concept*
    - A well-balanced diet using the MyPlate and a healthy weight are guidelines to prevent cancer.
      ○ Increase high-fiber plant-based foods.
      ○ Limit saturated and polyunsaturated fat, while emphasizing foods with monounsaturated fat or omega-3 fatty acids (nuts and fish).
      ○ Limit sodium intake.
      ○ Avoid excess alcohol intake.
      ○ Include regular physical activity.

    Ⓝ NCLEX® Connection: Health Promotion and Maintenance, Health Promotion/Disease Prevention

chapter 5

Overview

- Food safety is an important concept in nursing. It is essential to provide clients with the necessary education regarding food safety and food-medication interactions.

- Food safety concerns include preventing aspiration of food, reducing the risk of foodborne illness, assessing for food allergies, and understanding food-medication interactions.

Food Safety

- Ingestion of food poses a risk of aspiration in some circumstances.
  - To minimize the risk of aspiration, food should be consumed only by individuals who are conscious and have an intact gag or swallow reflex.
  - For clients who have a known risk of aspiration (following a stroke or a procedure involving anesthesia of the esophagus), it is important for nurses to monitor the client's ability to swallow prior to eating.

- Food safety requires:
  - Proper food storage.
  - Proper handling.
  - Proper preparation guidelines.

- Proper food storage guidelines
  - Fresh meat: 1 to 2 days at 40° F (4° C) or colder.
  - Fish: 1 to 2 days at 40° F (4° C) or colder.
  - Dairy products: Store in the refrigerator for 5 days for milk, and 3 to 4 weeks for cheese.
  - Eggs: Store in the refrigerator for 3 weeks in shell, and 1 week for hard-boiled.
  - Fruits and vegetables: Keep for 3 to 5 days. Citrus fruits and apples, 1 week or longer.
  - Pantry items: Store in a dry, dark place at room temperature.
  - Canned goods: Store 1 year or longer at room temperature.

- Proper handling
  - Wash hands and food preparation surfaces frequently, and before handling food.
  - Separate foods to avoid cross-contamination.

- Proper preparation guidelines
  - Cook food to the proper temperature (roasts and steaks, 145° F (63° C); chicken, 180° F (82° C); ground beef, 160° F (71° C).
  - Products that contain eggs must be cooked to 160° F (71° C).
- It is important to understand packaging labels.
  - Sell-by date is the final recommended day of sale.
  - Use-by date is how long the product will maintain top quality.
  - Expiration date is the final day the product should be used or consumed.

Foodborne Illness

- Foodborne illnesses occur due to improper storage of food products and unsafe handling. In order to decrease the incidence of foodborne illnesses, primary education should be conducted by nurses. Proper handing and preparation is simple and includes performing frequent hand hygiene. It is important to refrigerate food products when necessary, and to avoid cross-contamination when preparing food. Food should be heated to adequate temperatures to kill unwanted bacteria. These basic principles can prevent the occurrence of foodborne illnesses.
- Foodborne illnesses pose the greatest risk to children, older adults, and immunocompromised and pregnant clients.
- Common Foodborne Illnesses
  - Salmonella – Occurs due to eating undercooked or raw meat, poultry, eggs, fish, fruit, and dairy products. Common manifestations include headache, fever, abdominal cramping, diarrhea, nausea, and vomiting. This condition can be fatal.
  - Escherichia coli 0157:H7 – Raw or undercooked meat, especially hamburger, can cause this foodborne pathogen. Findings include severe abdominal pain and diarrhea.
  - Shigella – Poor personal hygiene and improper hand hygiene commonly cause Shigella. Food sources include dairy products and salads. Findings include diarrhea.
  - Listeria monocytogenes – Soft cheese, raw milk products, undercooked poultry, meat, seafood, and vegetables can cause the illness. Listeria monocytogenes causes significant problems for newborns, pregnant clients, and immunocompromised clients. Onset occurs with the development of a sudden fever, diarrhea, headache, back pains, and abdominal discomfort. It can lead to stillbirth or miscarriage in pregnant clients.

Food Allergies

- Nutritional assessments include identification of food allergies.
  - Milk, peanuts, fish, eggs, and wheat are the most commonly reported food allergies.
  - Common reactions and manifestations may include nausea, vomiting, dyspnea, itching, dizziness, and headache. Some reactions are severe and can cause anaphylaxis.

Food-Medication Interactions

- Foods and medications can interact in the body in ways that alter the intended action of medications. The composition and timing of food intake should be considered in relation to medication use.

- Foods can alter the absorption of medications.

  - Decreased absorption: Food can decrease the rate and extent of absorption.

    - Reducing the rate of absorption alters the onset of peak effects.

    - Reducing the extent of absorption reduces the intended effect of the medication.

- Some medications cause gastric irritation. It is important to take certain medications (ibuprofen [Advil, Motrin], some antibiotics, amoxicillin [Amoxil], and some antidepressants, bupropion [Wellbutrin]) with food to avoid gastric upset.

- Certain foods alter the metabolism/actions of medications.

  - Grapefruit juice interferes with the metabolism of many medications, resulting in an increased serum level of the medication.

  - Consumption of foods high in vitamin K (green leafy vegetables, eggs, liver) can decrease the anticoagulant effects of warfarin (Coumadin).

  - Foods high in protein, amino acids, and vitamin B_6 can increase the metabolism of the anti-Parkinson's medication levodopa (L-dopa, Sinemet), which decreases the duration of its therapeutic effects.

  - Licorice can cause hyperkalemia (elevated serum potassium). Excess ingestion can be dangerous for clients taking digoxin (Lanoxin), stimulant laxatives, some beta-blockers, ACE inhibitors, some calcium channel blockers, monoamine oxidase (MAO) inhibitors, and spironolactone.

  - Tyramine is a naturally occurring amine found in many foods that has hypertensive effects similar to other amines (norepinephrine). Tyramine is metabolized by MAO, and clients taking MAO inhibitors who consume foods high in tyramine may suffer a hypertensive crisis. Foods high in tyramine include aged cheese, smoked meats, red wines, and pickled meats.

  - Herbal supplements can cause potential interactions with prescribed medications. It is important that any herbal medication consumed by a client be discussed with the provider.

Nursing Assessments/Data Collection and Interventions

- Nursing assessments should include a complete dietary profile of the client, medications, herbal supplements, baseline knowledge about food safety, and food-medication interactions.

- Nursing interventions should include basic teaching about food safety, and the interactions between food and client medications.

APPLICATION EXERCISES

1. A nurse is providing teaching for a client who has a new prescription for warfarin (Coumadin). Which of the following foods should the nurse instruct the client to avoid?

    A. Spinach

    B. Grapefruit

    C. Peanuts

    D. Milk

2. A nurse is providing teaching to a client who has a new prescription for digoxin (Lanoxin). Which of the following food choices should be limited while taking this medication? (Select all that apply.)

    _____ A. Bananas

    _____ B. Celery

    _____ C. Baked potatoes

    _____ D. Tuna

    _____ E. Apples

3. A nurse is caring for a client who has a prescription for levodopa (Sinemet). Which of the following should the client limit in her diet?

    A. Tyramine

    B. Vitamin C

    C. Magnesium

    D. Vitamin B_6

4. A nurse is providing teaching to a client about food safety. What should be included in the teaching? Use the ATI Active Learning Template: Basic Concept to complete this item to include:

    A. Food Storage Guidelines: Describe four.

    B. Foodborne Illness: Describe three and how they are acquired.

APPLICATION EXERCISES KEY

1. A. **CORRECT:** Spinach is a green leafy vegetable that is high in vitamin K and decreases the anticoagulant effects of warfarin.

    B. INCORRECT: Grapefruit does not contain vitamin K but is high in vitamin C, which boosts the immune system.

    C. INCORRECT: Peanuts do not contain vitamin K but are high in protein, which boosts the immune system.

    D. INCORRECT: Milk does not contain vitamin K but is high in calcium, which promotes bone formation.

    Ⓝ NCLEX® Connection: Basic Care and Comfort, Nutrition and Oral Hydration

2. A. **CORRECT:** Bananas are high in potassium. Digoxin lowers serum potassium levels, and foods containing potassium should be encouraged.

    B. INCORRECT: Celery does not contain potassium and does not need to be limited while taking digoxin.

    C. **CORRECT:** Baked potatoes are high in potassium. Digoxin lowers serum potassium levels, and foods containing potassium should be encouraged.

    D. INCORRECT: Tuna is low in potassium and does not need to be limited while taking digoxin.

    E. INCORRECT: Apples are low in potassium and do not need to be limited while taking digoxin.

    Ⓝ NCLEX® Connection: Basic Care and Comfort, Nutrition and Oral Hydration

3. A. INCORRECT: Tyramine should be limited for a client who is taking a monoamine oxidase inhibitor, which increase blood pressure.

    B. INCORRECT: Vitamin C should be limited for a client taking proton pump inhibitors, which can affect the efficacy of this medication.

    C. INCORRECT: Calcium should not be limited unless the client is allergic to foods containing calcium.

    D. **CORRECT:** Vitamin B_6 should be limited while taking levodopa. Vitamin B_6 increases the metabolism of levodopa, which decreases the therapeutic effects of this medication.

    Ⓝ NCLEX® Connection: Basic Care and Comfort, Nutrition and Oral Hydration

4. *Using the ATI Active Learning Template: Basic Concept*

A. Proper Food Storage Guidelines
- Fresh meat: 1 to 2 days at 40° F (4° C) or colder.
- Fish: 1 to 2 days at 40° F (4° C) or colder.
- Dairy products: Store in the refrigerator for 5 days for milk, and 3 to 4 weeks for cheese.
- Eggs: Store in the refrigerator for 3 weeks in shell, and 1 week for hard-boiled.
- Fruits and vegetables: Keep for 3 to 5 days. Citrus fruits and apples, 1 week or longer.
- Pantry items: Store in a dry, dark place at room temperature.
- Canned goods: Store 1 year or longer at room temperature.

B. Foodborne Illnesses
- Salmonella – Occurs due to eating undercooked or raw meat, poultry, eggs, fish, fruit, and dairy products. Common manifestations include headache, fever, abdominal cramping, diarrhea, nausea, and vomiting. This condition can be fatal.
- Escherichia coli 0157:H7 – Raw or undercooked meat, especially hamburger, can cause this foodborne pathogen. Findings include severe abdominal pain and diarrhea.
- Shigella – Poor personal hygiene and improper hand hygiene commonly cause Shigella. Food sources include dairy products and salads. Findings include diarrhea.
- Listeria monocytogenes – Soft cheese, raw milk products, undercooked poultry, meat, seafood, and vegetables can cause the illness. Listeria monocytogenes causes significant problems for newborns, pregnant clients, and immunocompromised clients. Onset includes the development of a sudden fever, diarrhea, headache, back pains, and abdominal discomfort. It can lead to stillbirth or miscarriage in the pregnant client.

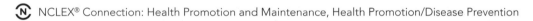 NCLEX® Connection: Health Promotion and Maintenance, Health Promotion/Disease Prevention

chapter 6

Overview

- Cultural, ethnic, and religious considerations greatly affect nutritional health. It is imperative that nurses gain a greater understanding of cultural needs.

- Cultural traditions impact food choices and routines. Nurses should consider these implications when planning and communicating nutritional goals with clients.

- Acculturation is the process of a cultural, ethnic, or religious group's adopting of the dominant culture's behaviors, beliefs, and values.

- Nurses must take care to avoid demonstrating ethnocentrism, which is the belief that one's own cultural practices are the only correct behaviors, beliefs, attitudes, and values.

Culture and Nutrition

- The degree to which clients follow their cultural, ethnic, or religious group's traditional nutritional practices should guide the nurse's care.

- The first generation members of a family are more likely to follow their traditional foodway (all aspects of an individual's nutritional practices), with subsequent generations incorporating the host culture's food practices through socialization.

- Frequently, the dominant culture's breakfast and lunch foods are eaten, and traditional meals are consumed at dinner and symbolic events (religious holidays, weddings, childbirth).

- To avoid ethnocentrism, nurses should understand that ideas regarding food choices and nutrition vary among cultures. For instance:

  ○ Beetles and bugs are food items in some cultures.

  ○ Not all cultures identify with the American ideal of slimness.

  ○ Milk is not a source of calcium in many cultures (especially when compared to the Euro-American foodway) due to the high incidence of lactose intolerance.

- Culturally respectful communication is necessary in all forms of client communication, including client education on nutrition.

  ○ The appropriateness of eye contact, touch, orientation to time ,and literacy vary among cultures and can impact communication.

  ○ Americanization of traditional foodways can have positive or negative consequences.

    ▪ New foods are added to the traditional diet.

    ▪ Food dishes are made in new ways.

    ▪ Cuisine items may be deleted entirely.

- Religion has a profound influence on foodways, especially because religion crosses geographic boundaries. Implications include:
  - Feasting/celebration foods.
  - Special food preparations (kosher kitchens in Orthodox Jewish homes).
  - Prescriptive guidelines for animal slaughter (Islam and Orthodox Judaism).
  - Avoidance of stimulants (coffee, tea, caffeinated soda) by Muslims and Mormons.
  - The practice of vegetarianism by Seventh-Day Adventists and some Buddhists.
  - Fasting for religious holidays (Ramadan for Muslims, or refraining from meat consumption on Ash Wednesday and Fridays during Lent for Catholics).
- Changes in the American foodway reflect cultural changes in American society and present nutritional challenges. Some trends that have made a significant impact on nutrition include:
  - Make it quickly.
  - Make it easy and add only three to four ingredients, or pop it ready-made into the microwave.
  - When all else fails, go to the drive-thru, order in, or eat out.
- Paying careful attention to reading labels, adding beneficial side dishes, practicing portion control, and choosing better dine-out options can minimize the detrimental effect of societal changes. These changes result in diets that are high in salt, carbohydrates, fat, refined sugars, and caffeine while providing low amounts of fiber and calcium.

Meeting Nutritional Needs with a Vegetarian Diet

- Individuals following a pure vegan diet do not consume animal products of any type, including eggs and milk products. These diets are often adequate in protein due to the intake of nuts and legumes (dried peas and cooked beans). Vitamin B_{12} and vitamin D supplementation may be needed with a pure vegan diet.
  - A pure vegan diet requires that a variety of plant materials be consumed in specific combinations in order to ensure essential amino acid intake.
- Individuals following a lacto vegetarian diet consume milk products in addition to vegetables.
- Individuals following a ovo-lacto vegetarian diet consume milk products and eggs in addition to vegetables.

Selected U.S. Cultural Subgroups

- African American ("Soul Food"): origins in the Caribbean, Central America, East Africa, and West Africa
  - Traditional foods
    - Rice, grits, cornbread; hominy, okra, greens, sweet potatoes; apples, peaches; buttermilk, pudding, cheddar or American cheese; ham, pork, chicken, catfish, black-eyed peas, red and pinto beans, peanuts; soft drinks, fatback, chitterlings, banana pudding
  - Traditional food preparation
    - Frying and cooking with added animal fats (lard, salt pork)
    - Promoting a shared inheritance and loving family

- ○ Acculturation
  - ▪ Increased milk consumption
  - ▪ Use of packaged meat, pork preferred
  - ▪ Continued low intake of fruit and vegetables
- ○ Nutritional health risks
  - ▪ High in fat, protein, and sodium, and low in potassium, calcium, and fiber
  - ▪ Low fresh fruit and vegetable intake
  - ▪ Substantial weight is equated with good health and prosperity
  - ▪ Increased incidence of type 2 diabetes mellitus and hypertension
- ○ Health promotion
  - ▪ Encourage frying lightly with canola/olive oil instead of animal fats.
  - ▪ Introduce fresh fruit and vegetable dishes and decrease meat portions.
  - ▪ Suggest dark green leafy vegetables and low-fat cheeses as calcium sources.
  - ▪ Associate "good health" with better food choices and portion control.
  - ▪ Advise preparing unhealthy soul food items only at special occasions.
- Asian American ("Chinese Food"): origins in the Far East, Southeast Asia, and the Indian subcontinent
  - ○ Traditional foods
    - ▪ Wheat (northern), rice (southern), noodles; fruits, land and sea vegetables, nuts/seeds, soy foods (tofu), nut/seed oils; fish, shellfish, poultry, eggs; sweets; rarely red meats; tea, beer
  - ○ Traditional food preparation
    - ▪ Fruits and vegetables peeled and raw
    - ▪ Stir-frying in oils quickly to retain crispness of vegetables
    - ▪ Cutting meat and poultry into bite-sized pieces
    - ▪ Cooking with salt, oil, and oil products (spices important)
    - ▪ Preventing imbalances and indigestion through balance of yin and yang
  - ○ Acculturation
    - ▪ Increased use of bread and cereal; rice/wheat staple remains high
    - ▪ Use of new location's fruit and vegetables with increased use of fruit and salads
    - ▪ Increased use of sugar through soft drinks, candy, and desserts
  - ○ Nutritional health risks
    - ▪ High sodium intake
    - ▪ Increased cancer rate as living in the U.S. continues
  - ○ Health promotion
    - ▪ Encourage continued use of plant-based diet and food preparation as generations take on "American foods."
    - ▪ Moderate salt intake.
    - ▪ Limit sugar-laden foods.

- Latino American ("Mexican Food"): origins in Mexico, Caribbean, and Central and South America
  - Traditional foods
    - Rice, maize, tortillas; tropical fruits, vegetables; nuts, beans, legumes; eggs, cheese, seafood, poultry; infrequent sweets and red meat
  - Traditional food preparation
    - Frying and stewing in lard or oil
    - Meats ground or chopped
    - Meat mixed with vegetables and grains, or stuffed (tamales)
    - Heavily spiced with common use of chilies
    - Minimal use of sugar
    - "Hot" and "cold" food choices maintain balance
  - Acculturation
    - Increased milk use
    - Decreased meat consumption as mixed meals decline
    - Replacement of maize by wheat in tortillas and breads
    - Decreased bean use and change in rice preparation to plain boiled rice
    - Increased fruit and vegetable intake
    - Added fats in the form of butter or salad dressings on cooked vegetables and side salads
    - Replacement of fruit-based drinks by sugar-laden drinks
  - Nutritional health risks
    - Increased incidence of type 2 diabetes mellitus
    - Positive associations with substantial weight
  - Health promotion
    - Encourage boiling, braising, and baking in place of frying and stewing in lard and oils.
    - Return to traditional corn tortillas.
    - Encourage use of fresh unprocessed/preserved plant-based diet.

APPLICATION EXERCISES

1. A nurse is providing teaching to a client about increasing calcium in the diet. Which of the following is an ethnocentric approach to selecting food choices on the client's menu to meet this need?

    A. Asking the client what he likes to eat

    B. Notifying the dietician to complete the menu

    C. Recommending one's own favorite foods

    D. Asking the client's family to fill out the menu

2. A nurse is caring for an Asian client who has hypertension. Which of the traditional Asian dietary patterns places the client at risk for this condition?

    A. Incorporation of plant based foods in the diet

    B. Consumption of raw fruits

    C. Preparation of foods using sodium

    D. A focus on shellfish in the diet

3. A nurse educator is teaching a class on culture and food to a group of newly hired nurses. Which of the following statements by the nurse indicates a need for clarification?

    A. "Clients who practice Roman Catholicism do not drink caffeinated beverages."

    B. "By working closely with nutrition services, nurses can meet the client's prescribed diet while promoting their religious practices."

    C. "Clients who follow the teachings of Islam eat only the protein of animals that are slaughtered under strict guidelines."

    D. "Because not all individuals in one country practice the same religion, a nurse should not consider ethnicity alone in planning for client care."

4. A nurse is completing an assessment of a client who is a first generation immigrant to the U.S. Which of the following questions should the nurse consider asking to understand the client's culture-based nutrition habits?

    A. "What type of afternoon snacks do you consume?"

    B. "What type of meal do you prepare for a holiday?"

    C. "What time of day do you eat breakfast?"

    D. "What cooking utensils are used in food preparation?"

5. A nurse is providing teaching to a Latin American client on nutrition. What should be reviewed in the teaching? Use the ATI Active Learning Template: Basic Concept to complete this item to include the following:

    A. Traditional Food Preparation: Describe four characteristics in the Latin culture.

    B. Acculturation: Describe three examples among Latinos living in the U.S.

    C. Health Risks: Describe two risks related to the Latin American diet.

APPLICATION EXERCISES KEY

1. A. INCORRECT: Asking the client what he likes to eat is not an example of an ethnocentric approach.

    B. INCORRECT: Calling the dietician to fill out the menu is not an example of an ethnocentric approach.

    C. **CORRECT:** Recommending one's own favorite foods is an example of ethnocentrism, which is the belief that one's own cultural practices are the only correct behaviors/beliefs.

    D. INCORRECT: Having the family fill out the menu is not an example of an ethnocentric approach.

    Ⓝ NCLEX® Connection: Psychosocial Integrity, Cultural Awareness/Cultural Influences on Health

2. A. INCORRECT: Plant-based foods are a good source of nutrition and should be encouraged.

    B. INCORRECT: The consumption of raw fruits is a good nutritional consideration related to increased vitamin intake and should be encouraged.

    C. **CORRECT:** The preparation of foods using sodium places the client at risk for hypertension. Many spices in the Asian diet contain sodium, or it is used as a preservative. Sodium consumption should be in moderation.

    D. INCORRECT: Consumption of shellfish is a good source of protein and vitamins and should be encouraged.

    Ⓝ NCLEX® Connection: Health Promotion and Maintenance, High Risk Behaviors

3. A. **CORRECT:** This is not a practice of Roman Catholics. Caffeinated beverages are not consumed by Mormons and Muslims because caffeine is a stimulant. This statement requires clarification.

    B. INCORRECT: This is an appropriate statement and does not require clarification.

    C. INCORRECT: This is an appropriate statement and does not require clarification.

    D. INCORRECT: This is an appropriate statement and does not require clarification.

    Ⓝ NCLEX® Connection: Health Promotion and Maintenance, High Risk Behaviors

4.   A. INCORRECT: This question considers acculturation patterns, not the client's cultural habits.

     B. **CORRECT:** Traditional meals are often consumed as part of the client's dinner or at symbolic events, such as holidays and weddings. This question helps the nurse understand culture-based nutrition habits.

     C. INCORRECT: This question does not incorporate culture-based dietary habits.

     D. INCORRECT: This question does not incorporate culture-based dietary habits.

     Ⓝ NCLEX® Connection: Psychosocial Integrity, Cultural Awareness/Cultural Influences on Health

5.   *Using the ATI Active Learning Template: Basic Concept*

     A. Traditional Food Preparation

        • Frying and stewing in lard or oil

        • Meats are ground or chopped

        • Meat is mixed with vegetables and grains, or stuffed (tamales)

        • Heavily spiced with common use of chilies

        • Minimal use of sugar

        • "Hot" and "cold" food choices maintain balance

     B. Acculturation

        • Increased milk use

        • Decreased meat consumption as mixed meals decline

        • Replacement of maize by wheat in tortillas and breads

        • Decreased bean use and change in rice preparation to plain boiled rice

        • Increased fruit and vegetable intake

        • Added fats in the form of butter or salad dressings on cooked vegetables and side salads

        • Replacement of fruit-based drinks by sugar-laden drinks

     C. Health Risks

        • Increased incidence of type 2 diabetes mellitus

        • Positive associations with substantial weight

     Ⓝ NCLEX® Connection: Psychosocial Integrity, Cultural Awareness/Cultural Influences on Health

UNIT 1   PRINCIPLES OF NUTRITION

CHAPTER 7   Nutrition Across the Lifespan

Overview

- Nutritional needs change as clients pass through the stages of the lifespan, reflecting physiological changes.

- Nurses must address nutritional needs across the lifespan and have a thorough understanding of how needs change. Nurses should focus on planning and implementing dietary plans that meet clients' specific needs.

- The major stages of the lifespan that have specific nutritional needs are:

  ○ Pregnancy and lactation

  ○ Infancy

  ○ Childhood

  ○ Adolescence

    ○ Adulthood and older adulthood

PREGNANCY AND LACTATION

Overview

- Prepregnancy nutrition is highly significant and plays an important role, because early fetal development occurs before a woman may realize she is pregnant. A woman should be well nourished and in her normal weight range prior to conception.

- Good nutrition during pregnancy is essential for the health of the unborn child.

- Maternal nutritional demands are increased for the development of the placenta, enlargement of the uterus, formation of amniotic fluid, increase in blood volume, and preparation of the breasts for lactation.

- A daily increase of 340 calories is recommended during the second trimester of pregnancy, and an increase of 452 calories is recommended during the third trimester of pregnancy.

- The nutritional requirements of women who are pregnant or lactating involves more than increased caloric intake. Specific dietary requirements for major nutrients and micronutrients should be taught.

Dietary Guidelines During Pregnancy and Lactation

- Achieving an appropriate amount of weight gain during pregnancy prepares a woman for the energy demands of labor and lactation, and contributes to the delivery of a newborn of normal birth weight.

- The recommended weight gain during pregnancy varies for each woman depending on her body mass index (BMI) and weight prior to pregnancy.

  o Recommended weight gain during the first trimester is 1 to 4 lb.

  o Recommended weight gain is 2 to 4 lb per month during the second and third trimesters.

  o Trimesters two and three:

    ▪ Normal weight client – 1 lb/week for a total of 25 to 35 lb.

    ▪ Underweight client – just more than 1 lb/week for a total of 28 to 40 lb.

    ▪ Overweight client – 0.66 lb/week for a total of 15 to 25 lb.

- Lactating women require an increase in daily caloric intake. If the client is breastfeeding during the postpartum period, an additional daily intake of 330 calories is recommended during the first 6 months, and an additional daily intake of 400 calories is recommended during the second 6 months.

Major and Micronutrient Requirements During Pregnancy and Lactation

- Dietary requirements for major nutrients

  o Protein should comprise 20% of the daily total calorie intake. The Dietary Reference Intake (DRI) for protein during pregnancy is 1.1 g/kg/day. Protein is essential for rapid tissue growth of maternal and fetal structures, amniotic fluid, and extra blood volume. Women who are pregnant should be aware that animal sources of protein might contain large amounts of fats.

  o Fat should be limited to 30% of total daily calorie intake.

  o Carbohydrates should comprise 50% of the total daily calorie intake. Ensuring adequate carbohydrate intake allows for protein to be spared and available for the synthesis of fetal tissue.

- The need for most vitamins and minerals increases during pregnancy and lactation. Vitamins are essential for blood formation, absorption of iron, and development of fetal tissue. The following table lists the comparative dietary reference intakes (DRIs) of major vitamins for women age 19 to 30 during nonpregnancy, pregnancy, and lactation.

DRIs OF MAJOR VITAMINS			
NUTRIENT	NONPREGNANT	PREGNANT	LACTATING
Protein (g)	46	71	71
Vitamin A (mcg)	700	770	1,300
Vitamin C (mg)	75	85	120
Vitamin D (mcg)*	15	15	15
Vitamin E (mcg)	15	15	19
Vitamin K (mcg)*	90	90	90
Thiamin (mg)	1.1	1.4	1.4

DRIs OF MAJOR VITAMINS			
NUTRIENT	NONPREGNANT	PREGNANT	LACTATING
Vitamin B_6 (mg)	1.3	1.9	2.0
Folate (mcg)	400	600	500
Vitamin B_{12} (mcg)	2.4	2.6	2.8
Calcium (mg)*	1,000	1,000	1,000
Iron (mg)	18	27	9

*Values represent adequate intakes (AIs).
Source: Office of Dietary Supplements. National Institutes of Health. Retrieved March 1, 2013, from ods.od.nih.gov

Additional Dietary Recommendations

- Fluid: 2,000 to 3,000 mL of fluids daily from food and drinks. Preferable fluids include water, fruit juice, or milk. Carbonated beverages and fruit drinks provide little or no nutrients.

- Alcohol: It is recommended that women abstain from alcohol consumption during pregnancy.

- Caffeine: Caffeine crosses the placenta and can affect the movement and heart rate of the fetus. However, moderate use (less than 300 mg/day) does not appear to be harmful.

- Vegetarian diets: Well-balanced vegetarian diets that include dairy products can provide all the nutritional requirements of pregnancy.

- Folic acid intake: It is recommended that 600 mcg/day of folic acid be taken during pregnancy. Current recommendations for lactating clients include 500 mcg/day of folic acid. It is necessary for the neurological development of the fetus and to prevent birth defects. It is essential for maternal red blood cell formation. Food sources include green leafy vegetables, enriched grains, and orange juice.

- Iron can be obtained from dairy products and meats, especially red meats. Consuming foods high in vitamin C aids in the absorption of iron.

Dietary Complications During Pregnancy

- Nausea and constipation are common during pregnancy.
  - For nausea, eat dry crackers or toast. Avoid alcohol, caffeine, fats, and spices. Avoid drinking fluids with meals, and do not take medications to control nausea without checking with the provider.
  - For constipation, increase fluid consumption and include extra fiber in the diet. Fruits, vegetables, and whole grains contain fiber.

- Maternal phenylketonuria (PKU) is a maternal genetic disease in which high levels of phenylalanine pose danger to the fetus.
  - It is important for a client to resume the PKU diet at least 3 months prior to pregnancy, and continue the diet throughout pregnancy.
  - The diet should include foods low in phenylalanine. Foods high in protein (fish, poultry, meat, eggs, nuts, dairy products) must be avoided due to high phenylalanine levels.
  - The client's blood phenylalanine levels should be monitored during pregnancy.
  - These interventions will prevent fetal complications (mental retardation, behavioral problems).

Nursing Assessments/Data Collection and Interventions

- Nursing assessments should include a complete profile of the client's knowledge base regarding nutritional requirements during pregnancy.
- Nurses should review the appropriate and recommended dietary practices for pregnant and lactating women with the client, while providing materials containing this information.

INFANCY

Overview

- Growth rate during infancy is more rapid than any other period of the life cycle. It is important to understand normal growth patterns to determine the adequacy of an infant's nutritional intake.
- Birth weight doubles by 4 to 6 months and triples by 1 year of age. The need for calories and nutrients is high to support the rapid rate of growth.
- Appropriate weight gain averages 0.15 to 0.21 kg (5 to 7 oz) per week during the first 5 to 6 months.
- An infant grows approximately 2.5 cm (1 in) per month in height the first 6 months, and approximately 1.25 cm (0.5 in) in height per month the last 6 months.
- Head circumference increases rapidly during the first 6 months at a rate of 1.5 cm (0.6 in) per month. The rate slows to 0.5 cm/month for months 6 to 12. By 1 year, head size should have increased by 33%. This is reflective of the growth of the nervous system.
- Breast milk, infant formula, or a combination of the two is the sole source of nutrition for the first 4 to 6 months of life. Currently, the American Academy of Pediatrics (AAP) recommends exclusive breastfeeding for the first 6 months of life, followed by breastfeeding with the introduction of complementary foods until at least 12 months of age, then continuation of breastfeeding for as long as the mother and infant desire.
- Semisolid foods should not be introduced before 4 months of age to coincide with the development of head control, ability to sit, and the back-and-forth motion of the tongue.
- Iron-fortified infant cereal is the first solid food introduced as gestational iron stores begin to deplete around 4 months of age.
- Cow's milk should not be introduced into the diet until after 1 year of age because protein and mineral content stress the immature kidney. A young infant cannot fully digest the protein and fat contained in cow's milk.

Meeting Nutritional Needs

- The American Academy of Pediatrics (AAP) recommends that infants receive breast milk for the first 6 to 12 months of age. Even a short period of breastfeeding has physiological benefits.

- The AAP recommends that for the first 6 months, infants should receive no water or formula except in cases of medical indication or informed parental choice. In the hospital, no water or formula should be given to a breastfed infant unless prescribed by a provider.

  ○ Advantages of breastfeeding

    ■ Incidence of otitis media (ear infections), type 1 and type 2 diabetes, obesity, leukemia, lymphoma, and gastrointestinal and respiratory disorders are reduced. This is due to the transfer of antibodies from mother to infant.

    ■ Carbohydrates, proteins, and fats in breast milk are predigested for ready absorption.

    ■ Breast milk is high in omega-3 fatty acids.

    ■ Breast milk is low in sodium.

    ■ Iron, zinc, and magnesium found in breast milk are highly absorbable.

    ■ Calcium absorption is enhanced as the calcium-to-phosphorous ratio is 2:1.

    ■ The risk of allergies is reduced.

    ■ Maternal-infant bonding is promoted.

  ○ Breastfeeding teaching points

    ■ The newborn is offered the breast immediately after birth and frequently thereafter. There should be eight to 12 feedings in a 24-hr period.

    ■ Instruct the mother to demand-feed the infant and to assess for hunger cues. These include rooting, suckling on hands and fingers, and rapid eye movement. Crying is a late sign of hunger.

    ■ The newborn should nurse up to 15 to 20 min per breast. However, avoid educating clients regarding an expected duration of feedings. Clients should be educated on how to evaluate when the newborn has completed the feeding by noting the slowing of newborn suckling, a softened breast, or sleeping.

    ■ Do not offer the newborn any supplements unless indicated by the provider.

    ■ The mother's milk supply is equal to the demand of the infant.

    ■ Eventually, the infant will empty a breast within 5 to 10 min, but may need to continue to suck to meet comfort needs.

    ■ Frequent feedings (every 2 hr may be indicated) and manual expression of milk to initiate flow may be needed.

    ■ If it has been 4 hr and the infant has not breastfed, the mother should awaken the infant for feeding.

    ■ Every effort will be made to encourage mothers to express breast milk for supplementation if extra fluids or calories are required.

    ■ Expressed milk can be refrigerated in sterile bottles or storage bags and labeled with the date and time the milk was expressed. It can be maintained in the refrigerator for 10 days or frozen in sterile containers for 6 months.

- Thaw milk in the refrigerator. It can be stored for 24 hr after thawing. Defrosting or heating in a microwave oven is not recommended because high heat destroys some of milk's antibodies, and may burn the infant's oral mucosa.

- Do not refreeze thawed milk.

- Unused breast milk must be discarded.

- Avoid consuming freshwater fish or alcohol, and limit caffeine.

- Instruct the mother to begin manual expression of her breast or use an electric breast pump if the infant is unable to breastfeed due to prematurity or respiratory distress.

- Do not take medications unless prescribed by a provider. The Infant Risk Center provides evidence-based information on the use of medications during pregnancy and lactation. Calls are answered Monday through Friday from 8 a.m. to 5 p.m. Central Standard Time at (806) 352-2519.

- Formula feeding
  - No artificial pacifier or bottles should be used until after 2 weeks and when breastfeeding is well established.

  - Commercial infant formulas provide an alternative to breast milk. They are modified from cow's milk to provide comparable nutrients. However, breast milk is far superior to any formula and even more crucial for a premature infant.

  - An iron-fortified formula is recommended by the American Academy of Pediatrics for at least the first 6 months of life or until the infant consumes adequate solid food. After 6 months, formula without added iron may be indicated.

  - Fluoride supplements may be required if an adequate level is not supplied by the water supply.

  - Wash hands prior to preparing formula.

  - Use sterile bottles and nipples.

  - Precisely follow the manufacturer's mixing directions.

  - Bottles of mixed formula or open cans of liquid formula require refrigeration. Do not use if the formula has been left at room temperature for 2 hr or longer. Do not reuse partially emptied bottles of formula.

  - Formula may be fed chilled, warmed, or at room temperature. Always give formula at approximately the same temperature.

  - Hold the infant during feedings with the head slightly elevated to facilitate passage of formula into the stomach. Tilt the bottle to maintain formula in the nipple and prevent the swallowing of air.

  - Do not prop the bottle or put an infant to bed with a bottle. This practice promotes tooth decay.

  - The infant should not drink more than 32 oz of formula per 24 hr period unless directed by a provider.

- Weaning
  - Developmentally, the infant is ready for weaning from the breast or bottle to a cup between 5 to 8 months of age.

  - If breastfeeding is eliminated before 5 to 6 months, a bottle should be provided for the infant's sucking needs.

  - It is best to substitute the cup for one feeding period at a time over 5 to 7 days.

  - Nighttime feedings are often the last to disappear.

○ Never allow a child to take a bottle to bed, as this promotes dental caries.

○ Use the new schedule for a second feeding period and continue at the infant's pace.

○ The infant may not be ready to wean from the bottle or breast until 12 to 14 months of age.

- Introducing solid food

  ○ Solid food should not be introduced before 4 to 6 months of age due to the risk of food allergies and stress on the immature kidneys. The AAP prefers introduction of solids foods after 6 months of age.

  ○ Indicators for readiness include voluntary control of the head and trunk, hunger less than 4 hr after vigorous nursing or intake of 8 oz of formula, and interest of the infant.

  ○ Iron-fortified rice cereal should be offered first. Wheat cereals should not be introduced until after the first year. Do not put cereal in the infant's bottle.

  ○ New foods should be introduced one at a time over a 4- to 5-day period to observe for signs of allergy or intolerance, which may include fussiness, rash, upper respiratory distress, vomiting, diarrhea, or constipation. Vegetables or fruits are first started between 6 and 8 months of age; after both have been introduced, meats may be added to the diet.

  ○ Delay the introduction of milk, eggs, wheat, and citrus fruits that may lead to allergic reactions in susceptible infants.

  ○ Do not give peanuts or peanut butter due to the risk of a severe allergic reaction.

  ○ The infant may be ready for three meals a day with three snacks by 8 months of age.

  ○ Homemade baby food is an acceptable feeding option. Do not use canned or packaged foods that are high in sodium. Select fresh or frozen foods, and do not add sugars or other seasonings.

  ○ Open jars of infant food may be stored in the refrigerator for up to 24 hr.

  ○ By 9 months of age, the infant should be able to eat table foods that are cooked, chopped, and unseasoned.

  ○ Do not feed the infant honey because of the risk of botulism.

  ○ Appropriate finger foods include ripe bananas, toast strips, graham crackers, cheese cubes, noodles, and peeled chunks of apples, pears, or peaches.

SUGGESTED INTRODUCTION OF FOODS	
Birth to 4 Months	› Breast milk (until 6 months) or formula (at 4 months)
4 to 6 Months	› Iron-fortified rice cereal
6 to 8 Months	› Vegetables, fruits
8 to 10 Months	› Strained meats, fish, poultry
9 to 12 Months	› Table foods (cooked, chopped, and unseasoned)
12 Months	› Cow's milk, eggs, cheese

Nutrition-Related Problems

- Colic is characterized by persistent crying lasting 3 hr or longer per day.
  - The cause of colic is unknown, but usually occurs in the late afternoon, more than 3 days per week for more than 3 weeks. The crying is accompanied by a tense abdomen and legs drawn up to the belly.
  - Colic usually resolves by 3 months of age.
  - Breastfeeding mothers should continue nursing, but limit caffeine and nicotine intake.
  - If breastfeeding, eliminating cruciferous vegetables (cauliflower, broccoli, and Brussels sprouts), cow's milk, onion, and chocolate may be helpful.
  - Burp the infant in an upright position.
  - Other comforting techniques (swaddling, carrying the infant, rocking, repetitive soft sound) may soothe the infant.
  - Most infants grow and gain weight despite colic.
  - Reassure the parent that colic is transient and does not indicate more serious problems or a lack of parental ability.
- Lactose intolerance is the inability to digest significant amounts of lactose (the predominant sugar of milk) and is due to inadequate lactase (the enzyme that digests lactose into glucose and galactose).
  - Lactose intolerance has an increased prevalence in individuals of Asian, Native American, African, Latino, and Mediterranean descent.
  - Clinical findings include abdominal distention, flatus, and occasional diarrhea.
  - Either soy-based (ProSobee or Isomil) or casein hydrolysate (Nutramigen or Pregestimil) formulas can be prescribed as alternative formulas for infants who are lactose intolerant.
- Failure to thrive is inadequate gains in weight and height in comparison to established growth and development norms.
  - Assess for clinical findings of congenital defects, central nervous system disorders, or partial intestinal obstruction.
  - Assess for swallowing or sucking problems.
  - Identify feeding patterns, especially concerning preparation of formulas.
  - Assess for psychosocial problems, especially parent-infant bonding.
  - Provide supportive nutritional guidance. Usually a high-calorie, high-protein diet is indicated.
  - Provide supportive parenting guidance.
- Diarrhea is characterized by the passage of more than three loose, watery stools over a 24-hr period.
  - Overfeeding and food intolerances are common causes of osmotic diarrhea.
  - Infectious diarrhea in the infant is commonly caused by rotavirus.
  - Mild diarrhea may require no special interventions. Check with the provider for any diet modifications.
  - Treatment for moderate diarrhea should begin at home with oral rehydration solutions (Pedialyte®, Infalyte®, ReVital®) or generic equivalents. After each loose stool, 8 oz of solution should be given. Sports drinks are contraindicated.
  - Educate parents about the clinical findings of dehydration: listlessness, sunken eyes, sunken fontanels, decreased tears, dry mucous membranes, and decreased urine output.

- ○ Breastfed infants should continue nursing.
- ○ Formula-fed infants usually do not require diluted formulas or special formulas.
- ○ Contact the provider if clinical findings of dehydration are present, or if vomiting, bloody stools, high fever, change in mental status, or refusal to take liquids occurs.
- Constipation is the inability or difficulty to evacuate the bowels.
  - ○ Constipation is not a common problem for breastfed infants.
  - ○ Constipation may be caused by formula that is too concentrated or by inadequate carbohydrate intake.
  - ○ Stress the importance of accurate dilution of formula.
  - ○ Advise adherence to the recommended amount of formula intake for age.

Nursing Assessments/Data Collection and Interventions

- Nursing assessments should include an assessment of knowledge base of the client regarding nutritional guidelines for infants, normal infant growth patterns, breastfeeding, formula feeding, and the progression for the introduction of solid foods.
- Additionally, nurses should provide education and references for the client regarding each of the assessments listed above.

CHILDHOOD

Overview

- Growth rate slows following infancy.
- There are few standard diet plans now on My Plate compared to The Food Pyramid. "SuperTracker" can be used to create an individualized plan based on age, gender, and body composition.
- Energy needs and appetite vary with the child's activity level.
- Generally, nutrient needs increase with age.
- Attitudes toward food and general food habits are established by 5 years of age.
- Increasing the variety and texture of foods helps the child develop good eating habits.
- Foods like hot dogs, popcorn, peanuts, grapes, raw carrots, celery, peanut butter, tough meat, and candy may cause choking or aspiration.
- Inclusion in family mealtime is important for social development.
- Group eating becomes a significant means of socialization for school-age children.
- ChooseMyPlate.gov, developed by the United States Department of Agriculture (USDA), is the recommended guide for providing adequate nutrition. Children require the same food groups as adults, but in smaller serving sizes.

Toddlers: 1 to 3 years old

- Nutrition Guidelines
  - Toddlers generally grow 2 to 3 inches in height and gain approximately 5 lb annually.
  - Limit 100% juice to 4 to 6 oz a day.
  - The 1- to 2-year-old child requires whole cow's milk to provide adequate fat for the still-growing brain.
  - Food serving size is 1 tbsp for each year of age.
  - Exposure to a new food may need to occur 8 to 15 times before the child develops an acceptance of it.
  - If there is a negative family history for allergies, cow's milk, chocolate, citrus fruits, egg white, seafood, and nut butters may be gradually introduced while monitoring the child for reactions.
  - Toddlers prefer finger foods because of their increasing autonomy. They prefer plain foods to mixtures, but usually like macaroni and cheese, spaghetti, and pizza.
  - Regular meal times and nutritious snacks best meet nutrient needs.
  - Snacks or desserts that are high in sugar, fat, or sodium should be avoided.
  - Children are at an increased risk for choking until 4 years of age.
  - Avoid foods that are potential choking hazards (nuts, grapes, hot dogs, peanut butter, raw carrots, tough meats, popcorn). Always provide adult supervision during snack and mealtimes. During food preparation, cut small bite-sized pieces that are easier swallow, and to prevent choking. Do not allow the child to engage in drinking or eating during play activities or while lying down.

- Nutritional Concerns/Risks
  - Iron
    - Iron deficiency anemia is the most common nutritional deficiency disorder in children.
    - Lean red meats provide sources of readily absorbable iron.
    - Consuming vitamin C (orange juice, tomatoes) with plant sources of iron (beans, raisins, peanut butter, whole grains) will maximize absorption.
    - Milk should be limited to the recommended quantities (24 oz) because it is a poor source of iron and may displace the intake of iron-rich foods.
  - Vitamin D
    - Vitamin D is essential for bone development.
    - Recommended vitamin D intake is the same (5 mcg/day) from birth through age 50. Children require more vitamin D because their bones are growing.
    - Milk (cow, soy) and fatty fish are good sources of vitamin D.
    - Sunlight exposure leads to vitamin D synthesis. Children who spend large amounts of time inside (watching TV, playing video games) are at an increased risk for vitamin D deficiency.
    - Vitamin D assists in the absorption of calcium into the bones.

Preschoolers: 3 to 6 years

- Nutrition Guidelines
  - ○ Preschoolers generally grow 2 to 3 inches in height and gain approximately 5 lb annually.
  - ○ Preschoolers need 13 to 19 g/day of complete protein in addition to adequate calcium, iron, folate, and vitamins A and C.
  - ○ Preschoolers tend to dislike strong-tasting vegetables (cabbage, onions), but like many raw vegetables that are eaten as finger foods.
  - ○ Food jags (ritualistic preference for one food) are common and usually short-lived.
  - ○ MyPlate guidelines are appropriate, requiring the lowest number of servings per food group.
  - ○ Food patterns and preferences are first learned from the family, and peers begin influencing preferences and habits at around 5 years of age.
- Nutritional Concerns/Risks
  - ○ Concerns include overfeeding; intake of high-calorie, high-fat, high-sodium snacks, soft drinks, and juices; and inadequate intake of fruits and vegetables.
    - Be alert to the appropriate serving size of foods (1 tbsp per year of age).
    - Avoid high-fat and high-sugar snacks.
    - Encourage daily physical activities.
    - May switch to skim or 1% low-fat milk after 2 years of age.
  - ○ Iron deficiency anemia (see previous information for toddlers).
  - ○ Lead poisoning is a risk for children under 6 years of age because they frequently place objects in their mouths that may contain lead, and have a higher rate of intestinal absorption.
    - Feed children at frequent intervals because more lead is absorbed on an empty stomach.
    - Inadequate intake of calories, calcium, iron, zinc, and phosphorous may increase susceptibility.

School-Age Children: 6 to 12 years

- Nutrition Guidelines
  - ○ School-age children generally grow 2 to 3 inches in height and gain approximately 5 lb annually.
  - ○ Following MyPlate recommendations, the diet should provide variety, balance, and moderation.
  - ○ Young athletes need to meet energy, protein, and fluid needs.
  - ○ Educate children to make healthy food selections.
  - ○ Children enjoy learning how to safely prepare nutritious snacks.
  - ○ Children need to learn to eat snacks only when hungry, not when bored or inactive.
- Nutrition Concerns/Risks
  - ○ Skipping breakfast occurs in about 10% of children.
    - Optimum performance in school is dependent on a nutritious breakfast.
    - Children who regularly eat breakfast tend to have an age appropriate BMI.

○ Overweight/obesity affects at least 20% of children.

- Greater psychosocial implications exist for children than adults.

- Overweight children tend to be obese adults.

- Prevention is essential. Encourage healthy eating habits, decrease fats and sugars (empty-calorie foods), and increase the level of physical activity.

- A weight-loss program directed by a provider is indicated for children who are more than 40% overweight.

- Praise the child's abilities and skills.

- Never use food as a reward or punishment.

Nursing Assessments/Data Collection and Interventions

- Nursing assessments should include the parent's knowledge base of the child's nutritional requirements, and nutritional concerns with regard to age. Nurses should provide education for the parent and child about nutritional recommendations.

ADOLESCENCE

Overview

- The rate of growth during adolescence is second only to the rate in infancy. Nutritional needs for energy, protein, calcium, iron, and zinc increase at the onset of puberty and the growth spurt.

- The female adolescent growth spurt usually begins at 10 or 11 years of age, peaks at 12 years, and is completed by 17 years. Female energy requirements are less than that of males, as they experience less growth of muscle and bone tissue and more fat deposition.

- The male adolescent growth spurt begins at 12 or 13 years of age, peaks at 14 years, and is completed by 21 years.

- Eating habits of adolescents are often inadequate in meeting recommended nutritional intake goals.

Nutritional Considerations

- Energy requirements average 2,000 cal/day for a 15-year-old female, and 4,000 cal/day for a 15-year-old male.

- The USDA reports that the average U.S. adolescent consumes a diet deficient in folate, vitamins A and E, iron, zinc, magnesium, calcium, and fiber. This trend is more pronounced in females than males.

- Diets of adolescents generally exceed recommendations for total fat, saturated fat, cholesterol, sodium, and sugar.

Nutritional Risks

- Eating and snacking patterns promote essential nutrient deficiencies (calcium, vitamins, iron, fiber) and overconsumption of sugars, fat, and sodium.

  ○ Adolescents tend to skip meals, especially breakfast, and eat more meals away from home.

  ○ Foods are often selected from vending machines, convenience stores, and fast food restaurants. These foods are typically high in fat, sugar, and sodium.

  ○ Carbonated beverages may replace milk and fruit juices in the diet with resulting deficiencies in vitamin C, riboflavin, phosphorous, and calcium.

- Adolescents have an increased need for iron.

  ○ Females 14 to 18 years of age require 15 mg of iron to support expansion of blood volume and blood loss during menstruation.

  ○ Males 14 to 18 years of age require 11 mg of iron to support expansion of muscle mass and blood volume.

- Inadequate calcium intake may predispose the adolescent to osteoporosis later in life.

  ○ During adolescence, 45% of bone mass is added.

  ○ Normal blood-calcium levels are maintained by drawing calcium from the bones if calcium intake is low.

  ○ Adolescents require at least 1,300 mg of calcium a day, which may be achieved by three to four servings from the dairy food group.

- Dieting

  ○ The stigma of obesity and social pressure to be thin can lead to unhealthy eating practices and poor body image, especially in females.

  ○ Males are more susceptible to using supplements and high-protein drinks in order to build muscle mass and improve athletic performance. Some athletes restrict calories to maintain or achieve a lower weight.

  ○ Eating disorders may follow self-imposed crash diets for weight loss.

- Eating disorders (anorexia nervosa, bulimia nervosa, obesity) are on the rise among adolescent clients. These disorders are discussed further in ATI Mental Health Nursing Review Module: Chapter 18.

- Adolescent Pregnancy

  ○ The physiologic demands of a growing fetus compromise the adolescent's needs for her own unfinished growth and development.

  ○ Inconsistent eating and poor food choices place the adolescent at risk for anemia, pregnancy-induced hypertension, gestational diabetes, premature labor, spontaneous abortion, and delivery of a newborn of low birth weight.

Nursing Assessments/Data Collection and Interventions

- Nursing assessments should include a determination of the adolescent's
  - Typical 24-hr food intake.
  - Weight patterns, current weight, and ideal body weight.
  - Attitude about current weight.
  - Use of nutritional supplements, vitamins, and minerals.
  - Medical history and use of prescription medications.
  - Use of over-the-counter medications, street drugs, alcohol, and tobacco.
  - Level of daily physical activity.
- Nurses should assess for clinical findings of an eating disorder. This may include an evaluation of the adolescent's laboratory values.
- Nursing assessments should include strategies that promote health for the adolescent.
  - Educate the adolescent on using MyPlate to meet energy and nutrient needs with three regular meals and snacks.
  - Stress the importance of meeting calcium needs by including low-fat milk, yogurt, and cheese in the diet.
  - Educate the adolescent on how to select and prepare nutrient-dense snack foods: unbuttered, unsalted popcorn; pretzels; fresh fruit; string cheese; smoothies made with low-fat yogurt, skim milk, or reduced-calorie fruit juice; and raw vegetables with low-fat dips.
  - Encourage participation in vigorous physical activity at least three times a week.
  - Refer pregnant adolescents to the Women, Infant, and Children (WIC) nutrition subsidy program.
  - Provide individual and group counseling for teens with clinical findings of eating disorders.

ADULTHOOD AND OLDER ADULTHOOD

Overview

- Nurses should assess the nutritional, physical, and mental health of adults and older adults.
- A balanced diet for all adults consists of 40% to 55% carbohydrate and 10% to 20% fat (with no more than 30% fat).
- The recommended amount for protein is unchanged in adults and older adults. However, many nutrition experts believe that protein requirements increase in older adults.
- Older adults need to reduce total caloric intake. This is due to the decrease in basal metabolic rate that occurs from the decrease in lean body mass that develops with aging.
- Reduced caloric intake predisposes the older adult for development of nutrient deficiencies.
- Regular exercise is encouraged for all adults.
- Older adults may have physical, mental, and social changes that affect their ability to purchase, prepare, and digest foods and nutrients.
- Dehydration is the most common fluid and electrolyte imbalance in older adults. Fluid needs increase with medication-induced fluid losses. Some disease processes necessitate fluid restrictions.

Nutritional Concerns

- A 24-hr dietary intake is helpful in determining the need for dietary education.

- Older adults may have oral problems (ill-fitting dentures, difficulty chewing or swallowing), and a decrease in salivation or poor dental health.

- Older adults have decreased cellular function and reduced body reserves, leading to decreased absorption of B_{12}, folic acid, and calcium, as well as reductions in insulin production and sensitivity.

- Decreased elasticity of blood vessels can lead to hypertension.

- Kidneys (renal) regulate the amount of potassium and sodium in the blood stream. Renal function can decrease as much as 50% in older adults.

- Older adults have a decreased lean muscle mass. Exercise can help to counteract muscle mass loss.

- The loss of calcium can result in decreased bone density in older adults.

- Cell-mediated immunity decreases as an individual ages.

Balanced Diet and Nutrient Needs

- MyPlate, developed by the USDA, suggests the following daily food intake for adults and older adults who get less than 30 min of moderate physical activity most days.

MYPLATE RECOMMENDATIONS FOR ADULTS						
	MEN			**WOMEN**		
	19 to 30	31 to 50	51+	19 to 30	31 to 50	51+
Calories	2,400	2,200	2,000	2,000	1,800	1,600
Fruits	2 cups	2 cups	2 cups	2 cups	1 ½ cups	1 ½ cups
Vegetables	3 cups	3 cups	2 ½ cups	2 ½ cups	2 ½ cups	2 cups
Grains	8 oz	7 oz	6 oz	6 oz	6 oz	5 oz
Meats and beans	6 ½ oz	6 oz	5 ½ oz	5 ½ oz	5 oz	5 oz
Milk	3 cups	3 cups	3 cups	3 cups	3 cups	3 cups
Oils	7 tsp	6 tsp	6 tsp	6 tsp	5 tsp	5 tsp

Source: United States Department of Agriculture. *ChooseMyPlate.gov*. Retrieved March 1, 2013, from www.choosemyplate.gov

- Grains: Select whole grains.
- Vegetables: Select orange and dark green leafy vegetables.
- Fruits: Select fresh, dried, canned, or juices. Avoid fruits with added sugar.
  - Make half your plate vegetables and fruits.
- Milk, yogurt, and cheese group: One cup of milk or plain yogurt is equivalent to 1 ½ oz of natural cheese or 2 oz processed cheese.
- Meat and bean group: Includes meat, fish, poultry, dry beans, eggs, and nuts. One ounce equals 1 oz meat, fish, or poultry (baked, grilled, broiled); ¼ cup cooked dry beans; 1 egg; 1 tbsp peanut butter; or ½ oz nuts. Use lean meats.

- Oils: Use vegetable oils (except palm and coconut). One tbsp of oil equals 3 tsp equivalent; 1 tbsp mayonnaise equals 2 ½ tsp dietary intake; and 1 oz nuts equals 3 tsp oils (except hazelnut, which equals 4 tsp).

- Discretionary calories: 132 to 362 discretionary calories are permitted per day. These add up quickly and can be from more than one food group.

- Minerals: Calcium requirements increase for older adults as the efficiency of calcium absorption decreases with age.

 - Vitamins: Vitamins A, D, C, E, B_6, and B_{12} may be decreased in older adults. Supplemental vitamins are recommended.

Regular Exercise

- All adults should exercise at a moderate or vigorous pace for at least 30 min per day, 3 to 7 days a week.

- Physical activity must increase heart rate to be relevant. Moderate activities include gardening/yard work, golf, dancing, and walking briskly.

- The loss of lean muscle mass is part of normal aging and can be decreased with regular exercise. The loss of lean muscle may be associated with a decrease in total protein and insulin sensitivity.

- Regular exercise can improve bone density, relieve depression, and enhance cardiovascular and respiratory function.

Potential Impact of Physical, Mental, and Social Changes

- Diseases and treatments may interfere with nutrient and food absorption, and utilization.

 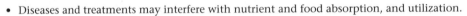
  - Aging adults are at an increased risk for developing osteoporosis (decreasing total bone mass and deterioration of bone tissue). Adequate calcium and vitamin D intake with regular weight-bearing exercise is important for maximizing bone density.

  - Osteoarthritis (OA) causes significant disability and pain in older adult clients. OA can limit mobility and present difficulty in obtaining and preparing proper foods.

  - Arthritis can interfere with the purchase and preparation of foods.

  - Alzheimer's disease is a form of dementia commonly seen in clients age 65 and older. This form of dementia causes impairments in memory and judgment that may make shopping, storing, and cooking food difficult.

- Certain medications (diuretics) for hypertension can cause sodium or potassium losses.

- Loss of smell and vision interfere with the interest in eating food.

- BMI should be between 18.5 and 24.9. There is an increased risk for both overweight and underweight older adult clients. Overweight adults are more prone to hypertension, diabetes, and cardiovascular events.

- Older adults may have difficulty chewing, in which case mincing or chopping food is helpful. They may have difficulty swallowing food, and thickened liquids may decrease the risk for aspiration.

- Social isolation, loss of a spouse, and mental deterioration may cause poor nutrition in adult and older adult clients. Encourage socialization and refer to a senior center or program.

- A fixed income may make it difficult for older adults to purchase needed foods. Refer to food programs, senior centers, and food banks. The Meals on Wheels program is available for housebound older adults.

Fluid Intake

- The long-held standard of consuming eight 8-oz glasses of liquid per day has been tempered by evidence that dehydration is not imminent even when less than 64 oz of fluid is consumed.

- Solid foods provide varying amounts of water, making it possible to get adequate fluid despite low beverage intake.

- For healthy adults, it is generally acceptable to allow normal drinking and eating habits to provide needed fluids.

- Encourage water and natural juices, and discourage drinking only soda pop and other liquids that have caffeine.

Nursing Assessments/Data Collection and Interventions

- Nursing assessments should include a dietary profile of the adult or older adult. Medical history, medication regimen, mobility, social practices, mental status, and financial circumstances are important components of the assessment. Nurses should provide education about proper dietary practices for the adult and older adult, while additionally providing referrals to community agencies when appropriate.

APPLICATION EXERCISES

1. A community nurse is providing education to a group of adult clients regarding exercise. Which of the following statements by a client indicates a need for additional teaching?

    A. "Regular exercise will improve my bone density."

    B. "Regular exercise can improve my cardiovascular health."

    C. "Regular exercise will regulate my menstrual cycle."

    D. "Regular exercise can relieve my depression."

2. A nurse in an assisted living facility is caring for an older adult client. The nurse should recognize that older adults have decreased absorption of which of the following? (Select all that apply.)

    _____ A. Calcium

    _____ B. Chloride

    _____ C. Folic acid

    _____ D. Magnesium

    _____ E. Phosphorus

3. A nurse in an antepartum clinic is discussing with a newly licensed nurse poor nutrition and risk for pregnant adolescent clients. Which of the following statements by the newly licensed nurse requires additional teaching?

    A. "Pregnant adolescents are at risk for having a placenta previa."

    B. "Pregnant adolescents are at risk for developing gestational diabetes."

    C. "Pregnant adolescents are at risk for having a low birth weight baby."

    D. "Pregnant adolescents are at risk for developing pregnancy-induced hypertension."

4. A nurse is discussing clinical findings of dehydration in an infant with a newly licensed nurse. Which of the following statements by the newly licensed nurse requires additional teaching?

    A. "The infant may appear listless."

    B. "The infant will have decreased urinary output."

    C. "The infant will have bulging fontanels."

    D. "The infant will have dry mucous membranes."

5. A nurse is assessing a 6-month-old infant who has a lactose intolerance. Which of the following clinical findings are associated with this diagnosis? (Select all that apply.)

_____ A. Abdominal distention

_____ B. Flatus

_____ C. Hypoactive bowel sounds

_____ D. Occasional diarrhea

_____ E. Visible peristalsis

6. A nurse is providing nutritional education to the parents of a toddler. Which of the following statements by the parents requires additional teaching?

A. "I should give my child finger foods."

B. "I should limit juice to 8 ounces daily."

C. "My child's serving size should be 1 tablespoon for each year of age."

D. "My child should gain about 5 pounds this year."

7. A nurse is teaching the parents of a toddler about appropriate snack foods. Which of the following should be included in the teaching? (Select all that apply.)

_____ A. Graham crackers

_____ B. Apple slices

_____ C. Peeled raisins

_____ D. Jelly beans

_____ E. Cheese cubes

8. A nurse is teaching a nutritional class for a group of pregnant clients. Which of the following should be included in the teaching regarding iron-rich foods? (Select all that apply.)

_____ A. Beans

_____ B. Fish

_____ C. Diary products

_____ D. Lean red meats

_____ E. Apples

9. A school nurse is conducting a nutrition course to a group of teens. Which of the following should be included as healthy snack choices? (Select all that apply.)

_____ A. Carrot sticks with low-fat dip

_____ B. Cheese and crackers

_____ C. Unbuttered popcorn

_____ D. Frozen low-fat yogurt

_____ E. Hot dog

10. A nurse is reviewing prescribed medications for an older adult client. Which of the following medications could result in sodium and potassium loss?

A. Hydrochlorothiazide (HydroDIURIL)

B. Captopril (Capoten)

C. Guaifenesin (Anti-Tuss)

D. Cephalexin (Keflex)

11. A community health nurse is teaching a group of parents the importance of adequate vitamin D intake for children. Use the ATI Active Learning Template: Basic Concept to complete this item to name two sources of vitamin D.

APPLICATION EXERCISES KEY

1. A. INCORRECT: Regular weight-bearing exercise is important for maximizing bone density, so this statement does not indicate a need for additional teaching.

    B. INCORRECT: Regular exercise can enhance cardiovascular health, so this statement does not indicate a need for additional teaching.

    C. **CORRECT:** Regular exercise does not regulate the menstrual cycle. This statement requires additional teaching.

    D. INCORRECT: Regular exercise can assist in decreasing depression, so this statement does not indicate a need for additional teaching.

    Ⓝ NCLEX® Connection: Health Promotion and Maintenance, Health Promotion/Disease Prevention

2. A. **CORRECT:** Older adults have decreased cellular function and reduced body reserves, leading to decreased absorption of B_{12}, folic acid, and calcium.

    B. INCORRECT: Older adults do not have decreased absorption of chloride.

    C. **CORRECT:** Older adults have decreased cellular function and reduced body reserves, leading to decreased absorption of B_{12}, folic acid, and calcium.

    D. INCORRECT: Older adults do not have decreased absorption of magnesium.

    E. INCORRECT: Older adults do not have decreased absorption of phosphorus.

    Ⓝ NCLEX® Connection: Health Promotion and Maintenance, Aging Process

3. A. **CORRECT:** Poor nutritional status does not place the adolescent client at risk for having a placenta previa. This statement requires additional teaching.

    B. INCORRECT: Inconsistent eating and poor food choices place the adolescent at risk for anemia, pregnancy-induced hypertension, gestational diabetes, premature labor, spontaneous abortion, and delivery of a newborn of low birth weight.

    C. INCORRECT: Inconsistent eating and poor food choices place the adolescent at risk for anemia, pregnancy-induced hypertension, gestational diabetes, premature labor, spontaneous abortion, and delivery of a newborn of low birth weight.

    D. INCORRECT: Inconsistent eating and poor food choices place the adolescent at risk for anemia, pregnancy-induced hypertension, gestational diabetes, premature labor, spontaneous abortion, and delivery of a newborn of low birth weight.

    Ⓝ NCLEX® Connection: Health Promotion and Maintenance, Ante/Intra/Postpartum and Newborn Care

4. A. INCORRECT: Listlessness is a clinical finding associated with dehydration.

    B. INCORRECT: Decreased urinary output is a clinical finding associated with dehydration.

    C. **CORRECT:** Bulging fontanels are a clinical finding associated with increased intracranial pressure. This statement by the newly licensed nurse requires additional teaching.

    D. INCORRECT: Decreased tears and dry mucous membranes are clinical findings associated with dehydration.

    Ⓝ NCLEX® Connection: Basic Care and Comfort, Nutrition and Oral Hydration

5. A. **CORRECT:** Abdominal distention is a clinical finding associated with a lactose intolerance.

    B. **CORRECT:** Flatus is a clinical finding associated with a lactose intolerance.

    C. INCORRECT: Hypoactive bowel sounds are not associated with a lactose intolerance.

    D. **CORRECT:** Occasional diarrhea is a clinical finding associated with a lactose intolerance.

    E. INCORRECT: Visible peristalsis is not associated with a lactose intolerance.

    Ⓝ NCLEX® Connection: Health Promotion and Maintenance, Aging Process

6. A. INCORRECT: Toddlers prefer finger foods because of their increasing autonomy.

    B. **CORRECT:** Juice should be limited to 4 to 6 oz/day. This statement by the parents requires additional teaching.

    C. INCORRECT: Food serving size is 1 tbsp for each year of age.

    D. INCORRECT: Toddlers generally grow 2 to 3 inches in height and gain approximately 5 lb annually.

    Ⓝ NCLEX® Connection: Health Promotion and Maintenance, Aging Process

7. A **CORRECT:** Graham crackers are appropriate snack foods for toddlers.

    B. **CORRECT:** Apple slices are appropriate snack foods for toddlers.

    C. INCORRECT: Peeled raisins are difficult to chew and pose a choking hazard.

    D. INCORRECT: Jelly beans are difficult to swallow, pose a choking risk, and are high in sugar content.

    E. **CORRECT:** Cheese cubes are appropriate snack foods for toddlers.

    Ⓝ NCLEX® Connection: Health Promotion and Maintenance, Aging Process

8. A. **CORRECT:** Iron-rich foods include beans.

    B. **CORRECT:** Iron-rich foods include fish.

    C. **CORRECT:** Iron-rich foods include diary products.

    D. **CORRECT:** Iron-rich foods include lean red meats.

    E. INCORRECT: Apples are not rich in iron.

    Ⓝ NCLEX® Connection: Health Promotion and Maintenance, Ante/Intra/Postpartum and Newborn Care

9. A. **CORRECT:** Carrot sticks with low-fat ranch dip are a healthy snack selection.

    B. **CORRECT:** Cheese and crackers are a healthy snack selection.

    C. **CORRECT:** Unbuttered popcorn is a healthy snack selection.

    D. **CORRECT:** Frozen low-fat yogurt is a healthy snack selection.

    E. INCORRECT: Hot dogs are not a healthy food choice because they are high in sodium and fat.

    Ⓝ NCLEX® Connection: Health Promotion and Maintenance, Aging Process

10. A. **CORRECT:** Hydrochlorothiazide is a diuretic and can cause sodium and potassium loss.

    B. INCORRECT: Captopril is an antihypertensive and does not cause decreased sodium and potassium levels.

    C. INCORRECT: Guaifenesin is an expectorant and does not cause decreased sodium and potassium levels.

    D. INCORRECT: Cephalexin is a first-generation cephalosporin and does not cause decreased sodium or potassium levels.

    Ⓝ NCLEX® Connection: Physiological Adaptations, Fluid and Electrolyte Imbalances

11. *Using the ATI Active Learning Template: Basic Concept*
    - Vitamin D is essential for the development of healthy bones. It is important in children because their bones are newly formed and continually growing. Vitamin D aids in the absorption of calcium into the bones. Sunlight exposure, milk (cow's, soy), and fatty fish are sources of vitamin D.

    Ⓝ NCLEX® Connection: Health Promotion and Maintenance, Aging Process

UNIT 2   ## Clinical Nutrition

CHAPTERS

› Modified Diets
› Enteral Nutrition
› Total Parenteral Nutrition

NCLEX® CONNECTIONS

When reviewing the chapters in this unit, keep in mind the relevant sections of the NCLEX® outline, in particular:

Client Needs: Basic Care and Comfort

› Relevant topics/tasks include:

  » Nutrition and Oral Hydration

    › Consider the client's choices regarding meeting nutritional requirements and/or maintaining dietary restrictions, including mention of specific food items.

    › Provide client nutrition through continuous or intermittent tube feedings.

    › Evaluate side effects of client tube feedings and intervene, as needed.

chapter 8

Overview

- Therapeutic nutrition is the role of food and nutrition in the treatment of diseases and disorders.
- The basic diet becomes therapeutic when modifications are made to meet client needs. Modifications may include increasing or decreasing caloric intake, fiber, or other specific nutrients; omitting specific foods; and modifying the consistency of foods.
- Nurses should collaborate with the dietician for nutritional or dietary concerns.

Types of Therapeutic Diets

- Clear Liquid Diet
  - Consists of foods that are clear and liquid at room temperature.
  - Primarily consists of water and carbohydrates. This diet requires minimal digestion, leaves minimal residue, and is non-gas forming. It is nutritionally inadequate and should not be used long term.
  - Indications include acute illness, reduction of colon fecal material prior to certain diagnostic tests and procedures, acute gastrointestinal disorders, and some postoperative recovery.
  - Acceptable foods are water, tea, coffee, fat-free broth, carbonated beverages, clear juices, ginger ale, and gelatin.
  - Limit caffeine consumption, which can lead to increased hydrochloric acid and upset stomach.
- Full Liquid Diet
  - Consists of foods that are liquid at room temperature.
  - Offer more variety and nutritional support than a clear liquid diet and can supply adequate amounts of energy and nutrients.
  - Acceptable foods include all liquids on a clear liquid diet, all forms of milk, soups, strained fruits and vegetables, vegetable and fruit juices, eggnog, plain ice cream and sherbet, refined or strained cereals, and puddings.
  - Evaluate the need for high-protein and high-calorie supplements if this diet is used more than 2 to 3 days.
  - Indications include a transition from liquid to soft diets, postoperative recovery, acute gastritis, febrile conditions, and intolerance of solid foods.

  - Provides oral nourishment for clients having difficulty chewing or swallowing solid foods. Use cautiously with clients who have dysphagia (difficulty swallowing) unless liquids are thickened appropriately.
  - Contraindicated for clients who have lactose intolerance or hypercholesterolemia. Use lactose-reduced milk and dairy products when possible.
- Blenderized Liquid (Pureed) Diet
  - Consists of liquids and foods that are pureed to liquid form.
  - The composition and consistency of a pureed diet varies, depending on the client's needs.

- Modify with regard to calories, protein, fat, or other nutrients based on the dietary needs of the client.
- Adding broth, milk, gravy, cream, soup, tomato sauce, or fruit juice to foods in place of water provides additional calories and nutritional value.
- Each food is pureed separately to preserve individual flavor.
- Indications include clients who have chewing or swallowing difficulties, oral or facial surgery, and wired jaws.

- Soft (Bland, Low-Fiber) Diet
  - Contains whole foods that are low in fiber, lightly seasoned, and easily digested.
  - Food supplements or snacks in between meals add calories.
  - Food selections vary and can include smooth, creamy, or crisp textures. Fruits, vegetables, coarse breads and cereals, beans, and other potentially gas-forming foods are excluded.
  - Indications include clients transitioning between full liquid and regular diets, or those who have acute infections, chewing difficulties, or gastrointestinal disorders.

- Mechanical Soft Diet
  - A regular diet that is modified in texture. The diet composition is altered for specific nutrient needs.
  - Includes foods that require minimal chewing before swallowing (ground meats, canned fruits, softly cooked vegetables).
  - Excludes harder foods (dried fruits, most raw fruits and vegetables, foods containing seeds and nuts).
  - Indications include limited chewing ability; dysphagia, poorly fitting dentures, and clients who are edentulous (without teeth); surgery to the head, neck, or mouth; and strictures of the intestinal tract.

- Regular Diet (Normal or House Diet)
  - Indicated for clients who do not need dietary restrictions. The diet is adjusted to meet age specific needs throughout the life cycle.
  - Many health care facilities offer self-select menus for regular diets.

  - Modify the regular diet to accommodate individual preferences, food habits, and ethnic values.

Nursing Assessments/Data Collection and Interventions

- Ongoing assessment parameters include daily weights, ordered laboratory values, and an evaluation of a client's nutritional and energy needs and response to diet therapy.
- Observe and document nutritional intake. Perform a calorie count if needed to determine caloric intake and to evaluate adequacy.
- Provide education and support for diet therapy.
- A prescription for a diet as tolerated permits a client's preferences while taking into consideration the client's ability to eat. Assess the client for hunger, appetite, and nausea when planning the most appropriate diet, and consult with a dietician.
- Dietary intake is progressively increased (from nothing by mouth to clear liquids to regular diet) following a major surgery. Nurses should assess for the return of bowel function (as evidenced by auscultation of bowel sounds and the passage of flatus) before advancing a client's diet.
- Nurses can increase a client's satisfaction with a hospital diet through courteous delivery, assistance with the tray, displaying a positive attitude toward the diet, and providing education and explanation of the diet.

APPLICATION EXERCISES

1. A nurse is caring for a client following an appendectomy. The nurse verifies the postoperative prescription, which reads "discontinue NPO status; advance diet as tolerated." Which of the following are appropriate for the nurse to offer the client? (Select all that apply.)

_____ A. Applesauce

_____ B. Chicken broth

_____ C. Sherbet

_____ D. Wheat toast

_____ E. Cranberry juice

2. A nurse is caring for a client who is to receive a full liquid diet due to dysphagia. Which of the following nursing actions is the highest priority?

A. Add thickener to liquids.

B. Educate the client about acceptable liquids.

C. Perform a calorie count of consumed liquids.

D. Offer high-protein liquid supplements.

3. A nurse is performing dietary needs assessments for a group of clients. A blenderized liquid diet is appropriate for which of the following clients? (Select all that apply.)

_____ A. A client who has a wired jaw due to a motor vehicle crash

_____ B. A client who is 24 hr postoperative following temporomandibular joint repair

_____ C. A client who has difficulty chewing due to a traumatic brain injury

_____ D. A client who has hypercholesterolemia due to coronary artery disease

_____ E. A client who is scheduled for a colonoscopy the next morning

4. A nurse is assessing a client who is postoperative following a colon resection. Which of the following findings indicates that the client is ready to transition from NPO to oral intake?

A. Client report of hunger

B. Urinary output exceeding 30 mL/hr

C. Decrease in incisional pain

D. Passage of flatus

5. A nurse is assisting a client who has a prescription for a mechanical soft diet with food selections. Which of the following are appropriate selections by the client? (Select all that apply.)

_____ A. Dried prunes

_____ B. Ground turkey

_____ C. Mashed carrots

_____ D. Fresh strawberries

_____ E. Cottage cheese

6. A nurse is planning care for a client who is transitioning to a regular diet following an acute gastrointestinal infection. Use the ATI Active Learning Template: Basic Concept to complete this item to include the following sections:

A. Underlying Principles: Identify the indication for a regular diet.

B. Nursing Interventions:
- Identify at least two assessments that are appropriate to determine the need for dietary modifications to the regular diet.
- Identify at least two nursing actions that are appropriate to monitor the client's response to diet therapy.

APPLICATION EXERCISES KEY

1.   A. INCORRECT: Applesauce is appropriate once the client's diet begins to advance. It is not appropriate as an initial postoperative selection.

B. **CORRECT:** Chicken broth is a clear liquid, which is appropriate as an initial selection for a client who is postoperative.

C. INCORRECT: Sherbet is appropriate once the client's diet begins to advance. It is not appropriate as an initial postoperative selection.

D. INCORRECT: Wheat toast is appropriate once the client's diet begins to advance. It is not appropriate as an initial postoperative selection.

E. **CORRECT:** Cranberry juice is a clear liquid, which is appropriate as an initial selection for a client who is postoperative.

N NCLEX® Connection: Basic Care and Comfort, Nutrition and Oral Hydration

2.   A. **CORRECT:** The client's safety is the highest priority. Therefore, adding thickener to the liquids is the priority nursing action to reduce the risk for aspiration.

B. INCORRECT: It is appropriate to educate the client about acceptable liquids. However, this does not address the greatest risk to the client and is therefore not the highest priority nursing action.

C. INCORRECT: It is appropriate to perform a calorie count of consumed liquids. However, this does not address the greatest risk to the client and is therefore not the highest priority nursing action.

D. INCORRECT: It is appropriate to offer high-protein liquid supplements. However, this does not address the greatest risk to the client and is therefore not the highest priority nursing action.

N NCLEX® Connection: Reduction of Risk Potential, Potential for Complications of Diagnostic Tests/ Treatments/Procedures

3.   A. **CORRECT:** A blenderized liquid diet is appropriate for a client who has a wired jaw.

B. **CORRECT:** A blenderized liquid diet is appropriate for a client following oral surgery.

C. **CORRECT:** A blenderized liquid diet is appropriate for a client who has difficulty chewing.

D. INCORRECT: Hypercholesterolemia is a potential contraindication for a full liquid diet and does not indicate a need for a blenderized liquid diet.

E. INCORRECT: A client who is scheduled for a colonoscopy should receive a clear liquid, rather than a blenderized liquid, diet.

N NCLEX® Connection: Reduction of Risk Potential, Potential for Alterations in Body Systems

4.   A. INCORRECT: Reports of hunger do not indicate intestinal activity, which is necessary prior to transitioning a client from NPO to oral intake.

   B. INCORRECT: Adequate urinary output does not indicate intestinal activity, which is necessary prior to transitioning a client from NPO to oral intake.

   C. INCORRECT: A decrease in incisional pain does not indicate intestinal activity, which is necessary prior to transitioning a client from NPO to oral intake.

   D. **CORRECT:** The passage of flatus is an indicator of intestinal activity, which indicates the client is ready to transition to oral intake.

   Ⓝ NCLEX® Connection: Basic Care and Comfort, Elimination

5.   A. INCORRECT: Dried fruits are excluded from a mechanical soft diet due to potential chewing difficulty.

   B. **CORRECT:** Ground meats require minimal chewing before swallowing and are therefore appropriate for a mechanical soft diet.

   C. **CORRECT:** Mashed carrots require minimal chewing before swallowing and are therefore appropriate for a mechanical soft diet.

   D. INCORRECT: Fresh strawberries are excluded from a mechanical soft diet due to seeds and potential chewing difficulty.

   E. **CORRECT:** Cottage cheese requires minimal chewing before swallowing and is therefore appropriate for a mechanical soft diet.

   Ⓝ NCLEX® Connection: Basic Care and Comfort, Nutrition and Oral Hydration

6.   *Using the ATI Active Learning Template: Basic Concept*

   A. Underlying Principles
     • A regular diet is indicated for clients who do not need dietary restrictions.

   B. Nursing Interventions
     • Assessments to determine the need for dietary modification.
       ○ Individual preferences.
       ○ Food habits.
       ○ Ethnic values or practices.
     • Assessments to monitor the client's response to diet therapy.
       ○ Obtain daily weight.
       ○ Monitor laboratory values.
       ○ Monitor energy level.
       ○ Observe and document nutritional intake.
       ○ Evaluate understanding of diet therapy.

   Ⓝ NCLEX® Connection: Physiological Adaptations, Illness Management

chapter 9

Overview

- Enteral nutrition (EN) is used when a client cannot consume adequate nutrients and calories orally, but maintains a partially functional gastrointestinal system.

- EN is administered when a client has a medical condition (burns, trauma, radiation therapy or chemotherapy, liver or renal dysfunction, infection and inflammatory bowel disease) that hinders the client's nutritional status.

- EN is administered when a client is neuromuscularly impaired and cannot chew or swallow food.

- EN feeding or gavage feeding for an infant is used when an infant is too weak for sucking, unable to coordinate swallowing, and lacks a gag reflex.

- Gavage feeding is implemented to conserve energy when an infant is attempting to breast feed or bottle feed, but becomes fatigued, weak, or cyanotic.

- EN consists of blenderized foods or a commercial formula administered by a tube into the stomach or small intestine. Enteral feedings most closely utilize the body's own digestive and metabolic routes. EN can augment an oral diet or be the sole source of nutrition.

Enteral Feeding Routes

- A client's medical status and the anticipated length of time that a tube feeding will be required determine the type of tube used.
  - Transnasal tubes are short-term (less than 3 to 4 weeks).
    - Nasogastric (NG) tubes are passed through the nose to the stomach.
    - Nasointestinal tubes are passed through the nose to the intestine.
    - For an infant or child, a polyurethane or silicone small bore feeding tube is inserted in the right or left nare. This flexible tube may remain taped in place for up to 30 days.
    - Nasoduodenal or nasojejunal tubes are for infants or children at risk for aspiration and regurgitation. The child or infant who has head trauma, is receiving mechanical ventilation or has gastroparesis that requires continuous enteral feedings using a mechanical pump to regulate the hourly rate.

- An ostomy is a surgically created opening (stoma) made to deliver feedings directly into the stomach or intestines.

  - Gastrostomy tubes are endoscopically or surgically inserted into the stomach. A percutaneous endoscopic gastrostomy (PEG) tube is placed with the aid of an endoscope.

    - Gastrostomy tube feedings are generally well-tolerated because the stomach chamber holds and releases feedings in a physiologic manner that promotes effective digestion. As a result, dumping syndrome is usually avoided.

    - Children generally tolerate a skin-level gastrostomy tube, which is known as a low-profile gastrostomy device. It is more comfortable, allows for increased mobility, and is fully immersible in water. Checking for residual is more difficult with this device because of the close proximity of the button on the skin.

  - Jejunostomy tubes are surgically inserted into the jejunal portion of the small intestine (jejunum).

- Endoscopic or surgical placement is preferred when long-term use is anticipated, or when a nasal obstruction makes insertion through the nose impossible.

- Placement into the stomach stimulates normal gastrointestinal function.

Enteral Feeding Formulas

- Commercial products are preferred over home-blended ingredients because they provide a known nutrient composition, controlled consistency, and bacteriological safety.

- Standard and hydrolyzed formulas are the two primary types of enteral feeding formulas available. They are categorized by the complexity of the proteins included.

  - Standard formulas, also called polymeric or intact, are composed of whole proteins (milk, meat, eggs) or protein isolates.

    - These formulas require a functioning gastrointestinal tract.

    - Most provide 1.0 to 1.2 cal/mL, but are available in high-protein, high-calorie, fiber-enriched, and disease-specific formulas.

  - Hydrolyzed formulas, or elemental, are composed of partially digested protein peptides and are referred to as free amino acids.

    - These formulas are used for clients who have a partially functioning gastrointestinal tract, or those who have an impaired ability to digest and absorb foods (inflammatory bowel disease, short-gut syndrome, cystic fibrosis, pancreatic disorders).

    - Most provide 1.0 to 1.2 cal/mL. High-calorie formulas provide 1.5 to 2.0 cal/mL. Partially hydrolyzed formulas provide other nutrients in simpler forms that require little or no digestion.

- Tube feedings may be packaged in cans or prefilled bags.

  - Prefilled bags and administration tubing should be discarded every 24 hr or according to facility policy, even if they are not empty.

  - Cans may be used to add formula to a generic bag to infuse via a pump, or for feedings directly from a syringe.

- Factors to consider in determining an appropriate formula
  - ○ Caloric density determines the volume of the formula necessary to meet the caloric needs of a client (1.0 to 1.2 cal/mL)
  - ○ Water content in formulas with 1.0 cal/mL should be 850 mL of water. Higher-calorie formulas have lower water content. The client may need additional free water to meet hydration needs.
  - ○ Protein density refers to formulas that are whole protein. Hydrolyzed protein contains free amino acids, and partially hydrolyzed formulas contain protein that is broken down.
  - ○ Osmolality of the formula is determined by the concentration of sugars, amino acids, and electrolytes.
    - ■ Osmolality is increased if the formula contains more digested protein.
    - ■ Hydrolyzed or partially hydrolyzed (predigested) formulas are higher in osmolality than standard formulas. They are also lactose-free.
  - ○ Fiber and residue content
    - ■ Standard-intact formulas are blended foods, milk-based formulas, or lactose-free formulas.
    - ■ Standard formulas that are enriched with fiber are recommended for clients who have constipation or diarrhea to normalize bowel movements.
    - ■ Residual free formulas are recommended for clients who initially begin EN to minimize abdominal distention from increased flatus.
  - ○ The presence of other nutrients include fats and carbohydrates, which may be modified according to a client's disease processes (respiratory disease, malabsorption, diabetes, kidney disease).

Enteral Feeding Delivery Methods

- The delivery method is dependent on the type and location of the feeding tube, type of formula administered, and the client's tolerance.
  - ○ Continuous drip method – Formula is administered at a continuous rate over a 16- to 24-hr period.
    - ■ Infusion pumps help ensure consistent flow rates.
      - □ A continuous gavage feeding administered to an infant via an infusion pump tends to decrease the total milk fat concentration and is not recommended.
    - ■ This method is recommended for critically ill clients because of its association with smaller residual volumes, and a lower risk of aspiration and diarrhea.
    - ■ Residual volumes should be measured every 4 to 6 hr.
    - ■ Feeding tubes should be flushed with water every 4 hr to maintain patency.
    - ■ If the volume of gastric residual exceeds the volume of formula given over the previous 2 hr, it may be necessary to reduce the rate of feeding and return aspirated formula to the stomach.
  - ○ Cyclic feeding – Formula is administered at a continuous rate over an 8- to 16-hr time period, often during sleeping hours.
    - ■ Often used for transition from total EN to oral intake.
  - ○ Intermittent tube feeding – Formula is administered every 4 to 6 hr in equal portions of 200 to 300 mL over a 30- to 60-min time frame, usually by gravity drip.
    - ■ Often used for noncritical clients, home tube feedings, and clients in rehabilitation.

- ○ Bolus feeding – A variation of intermittent feeding using a large syringe attached to the feeding tube. A large volume of formula (500 mL maximum, usual volume is 250 to 400 mL) is administered over a short period of time, usually less than 15 min, four to six times daily.
  - ■ Bolus feedings are delivered directly into the stomach. They may be poorly tolerated and may cause dumping syndrome.
    - □ Dumping syndrome occurs due to rapid emptying of the formula into the small intestine, resulting in a fluid shift. Manifestations include dizziness, rapid pulse, diaphoresis, pallor, and light-headedness.
  - ■ Mother's breast milk is recommended for bolus feeding in infants.
    - □ The rate of the bolus feeding should be no more than 5 mL of breast milk or formula over 5 to 10 min for a premature infant, and 10 mL for an older infant or child, to prevent nausea and regurgitation.

Nursing Actions

- • Preparation of the Client
  - ○ Prior to instilling enteral feeding, tube placement should be verified by radiography. Aspirating gastric contents and measuring pH levels are not considered reliable methods of verifying placement.

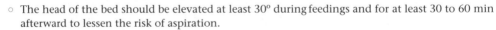

M View Video: Enteral Tube Feeding

  - ○ Verify the presence of bowel sounds.
  - ○ To maintain feeding tube patency, it is flushed routinely with warm water.
    - ■ Gastric residuals should be checked every 4 to 6 hr. If the residual volume exceeds the amount of formula given in the previous 2 hr, it may be necessary to consider reducing the rate of the feeding. Residuals should be returned to the stomach as they contain electrolytes, nutrients, and digestive enzymes. Follow facility policy.
      - □ For an infant – Subtract the amount of the residual from the amount of the formula to be given. Return the residual to the stomach plus the reduced amount of formula or breast milk.
      - □ For children – If the residual is more than one fourth of the previous feeding, return the residual to the stomach and recheck in 30 to 60 min.
      - □ Notify the provider if a large amount of residual continues to occur.

  - ○ The head of the bed should be elevated at least 30° during feedings and for at least 30 to 60 min afterward to lessen the risk of aspiration.
  - ○ Bubble the infant following the feeding if the infant's condition allows.
  - ○ Begin with a small volume of full-strength formula. Increase volume in intervals as tolerated until the desired volume is achieved.
  - ○ Administer the feeding solution at room temperature to decrease gastrointestinal discomfort.
  - ○ Do not heat formulas in a microwave as this can result in uneven temperatures within the solution.

- Baseline assessment parameters
  - Obtain height, weight, and body mass index (BMI).
  - Monitor serum albumin, hemoglobin, hematocrit, glucose, blood urea nitrogen (BUN), and electrolyte levels.
  - Evaluate the client's nutritional and energy needs.
  - Verify gastrointestinal function. Dysfunction of the gastrointestinal tract may indicate a need for alternate forms of nutrition.
- Ongoing Care
  - Monitor daily weights and I&O.
  - Obtain gastric residuals (every 4 to 6 hr).
  - Monitor electrolytes, BUN, creatinine, serum minerals, and CBC as prescribed.
  - Monitor the tube site for manifestations of infection or intolerance (pain, redness, swelling, drainage).
  - Monitor the character and frequency of bowel movements.
  - When appropriate, administer medications through a feeding tube.
    - Feeding should be stopped prior to administering medications.
    - The tubing should be flushed with water (15 to 30 mL) before and after the medication is administered, and between each medication if more than one is administered.
    - Liquid medications should be used when possible.
      - For an infant or child, the volume of water to flush is 1.5 times the amount predetermined to flush an unused feeding tube of the same size.
      - More water may be required to flush the tubing following certain medications (suspensions).
- Interventions
  - Weaning occurs as oral consumption increases. Enteral feedings may be discontinued when the client consumes two-thirds of protein and calorie needs orally for 3 to 5 days.

  - A client who is NPO will require meticulous oral care.
  - A client may require nutritional support service at home for long-term EN. A multidisciplinary team comprised of a nurse, dietician, pharmacist, and the provider, monitors the weight, electrolyte balance, and overall physical condition of the client.
  - Transitioning from EN to an oral diet requires the client to receive adequate nutrition as food items are reintroduced.
    - Begin the transition process by stopping the EN for 1 hr before a meal.
    - Slowly increase the frequency of the meals until the client is eating six small meals daily.
    - When oral intake equals 500 to 750 cal/day, the continuous tube feeding is administered only during the night.

Complications

- Gastrointestinal complications include constipation, diarrhea, cramping, pain, abdominal distention, dumping syndrome, nausea, and vomiting.
  - ○ Nursing Actions
    - ▪ Consider a change in formula.
    - ▪ Decrease the flow rate for the infusion.
    - ▪ Increase the volume of free water if constipated.
    - ▪ Administer the EN at room temperature.
    - ▪ Take measures to prevent bacterial contamination.
- Mechanical complications include tube misplacement or dislodgement; aspiration; tube obstruction or rupture; irritation and leakage at the insertion site; irritation of the nose, esophagus, and mucosa; and clogging of the feeding tube.
  - ○ Nursing Actions
    - ▪ Flush the tubing with 20 to 30 mL of warm water every 4 hr for continuous infusion, after returning residual formula into the stomach, and before and after bolus feedings and each medication administration.
    - ▪ Unclog tubing using gentle pressure with 50 mL of water in a piston syringe. Use carbonated beverage only when water does not open the tubing.
    - ▪ Do not mix medications with the formula.
- Metabolic complications include dehydration, hyperglycemia, electrolyte imbalances, and overhydration.
- Food poisoning can result due to bacterial contamination of formula.
  - ○ Nursing Actions
    - ▪ Prevent bacterial contamination.
      - ▫ Wash hands before handling formula or enteral products.
      - ▫ Clean equipment and tops of formula cans.
      - ▫ Cover and label unused cans with the client's name, room number, date, and time of opening.
      - ▫ Refrigerate unused portions promptly for up to 24 hr.
      - ▫ Replace the feeding bag, administration tubing, and any equipment used to mix the formula every 24 hr.
      - ▫ Fill generic bags with only 4 hr worth of formula.

APPLICATION EXERCISES

1. A nurse is discussing the use of a low-profile gastrostomy device with the parent of a child who is receiving an enteral feeding. Which of the following is an appropriate statement by the nurse?

   A. "The device can be uncomfortable for children."

   B. "Checking residual is much easier with this device."

   C. "Tub baths are allowed with this device."

   D. "Mobility of the child is limited with this device."

2. A nurse is teaching a client who is starting continuous feedings about the various types of enteral nutrition (EN) formulas. Which of the following should the nurse include in the teaching?

   A. Formula rich in fiber is recommended when starting EN.

   B. Standard formula contains whole protein.

   C. Hydrolyzed formula is recommended for a full-functioning GI tract.

   D. The high-calorie formula has increased water content.

3. A nurse is planning care for a client who is receiving continuous drip enteral nutrition. Which of the following interventions should be included in the plan of care? (Select all that apply.)

   _____ A. Administer with an infusion pump.

   _____ B. Measure residual every 8 hr.

   _____ C. Flush the feeding tube every 4 hr.

   _____ D. Reinstill the residual feeding into the stomach.

   _____ E. Reduce the flow rate if residual exceeds infused volume over the previous 3-hr period.

4. A nurse is administering bolus enteral feedings to a client who has malnutrition. Which of the following are appropriate nursing interventions? (Select all that apply.)

   _____ A. Verify the presence of bowel sounds.

   _____ B. Flush the feeding tube with warm water.

   _____ C. Elevate the head of the bed 20°.

   _____ D. Administer the feeding at room temperature.

   _____ E. Inspect the tube insertion site.

5. A nurse is preparing to administer intermittent enteral feeding to a client who has neuromuscular disorder. Which of the following are appropriate nursing interventions? (Select all that apply.)

_____ A. Fill the feeding bag with 24 hr worth of formula.

_____ B. Discard irrigation equipment after 24 hr.

_____ C. Leave unused portions of formula at the bedside.

_____ D. Label the unused portion of the formula.

_____ E. Replace administration tubing and feeding bag every 48 hr.

6. A nurse is providing information to a client on complications that can occur when administering an enteral nutrition. What information should the nurse include in the teaching? Use the ATI Active Learning Template: Basic Concept to complete this item to include the following:

A. Related Content:
- Identify three complications.
- List two nursing interventions for each complication.

APPLICATION EXERCISES KEY

1. A. INCORRECT: The gastrostomy device is more comfortable for children because of the close proximity of the button on the skin.

    B. INCORRECT: Checking for residual is more difficult with this device because of the close proximity of the button on the skin.

    C. **CORRECT:** The low-profile gastrostomy device is fully immersible in water.

    D. INCORRECT: The mobility of the child is decreased because of the close proximity of the button on the abdomen.

    Ⓝ NCLEX® Connection: Basic Care and Comfort, Nutrition and Oral Hydration

2. A. INCORRECT: Residual-free formula without fiber is recommended when starting EN to minimize abdominal distention from increased flatus.

    B. **CORRECT:** A standard formula contains whole protein (milk, meat, eggs) and requires a full-functioning GI tract.

    C. INCORRECT: Hydrolyzed formula is recommended for a partially functioning digestive tract or for those who have impaired ability to digest and absorb foods.

    D. INCORRECT: Formula high in calories is low in water content.

    Ⓝ NCLEX® Connection: Basic Care and Comfort, Nutrition and Oral Hydration

3. A. **CORRECT:** Administering continuous drip enteral nutrition using an infusion pump ensures the correct volume of the feeding is being infused.

    B. INCORRECT: The measurement of residual is preformed every 4 to 6 hr to determine if the formula is being digested.

    C. **CORRECT:** Flushing the feeding tube every 4 hr maintains patency.

    D. **CORRECT:** Reinstilling the residual feeding into the stomach returns needed fluids, electrolytes, nutrients, and digestive enzymes.

    E. INCORRECT: The flow rate should only be reduced if the residual volume of formula exceeds the amount administered over the previous 2 hr period.

    Ⓝ NCLEX® Connection: Basic Care and Comfort, Nutrition and Oral Hydration

4. A. **CORRECT:** The nurse should verify the presence of bowel sounds prior to a bolus feeding to ensure the bowel is functioning.

    B. **CORRECT:** The nurse should flush the feeding tube to ensure patency before administering a bolus feeding.

    C. INCORRECT: The nurse should elevate the client's head of bed at least 30° prior to a bolus feeding to decrease the risk of aspiration.

    D. **CORRECT:** The nurse should administer the bolus feeding at room temperature to prevent abdominal cramping.

    E. **CORRECT:** The nurse should inspect the tube site for manifestations of infection and leakage each time the client receives a bolus feeding.

    N NCLEX® Connection: Basic Care and Comfort, Nutrition and Oral Hydration

5. A. INCORRECT: The feeding bag should be filled with only enough formula for 4 hr to prevent bacterial contamination.

    B. **CORRECT:** Irrigation equipment should be discarded every 24 hr to prevent bacterial contamination.

    C. INCORRECT: The unused portion of formula should be refrigerated up to 24 hr to prevent bacterial contamination.

    D. **CORRECT:** The unused portion of the formula should be labeled with the time and date the formula was opened and the client's name and room number.

    E. **CORRECT:** Replace the administration tubing and feeding bag every 24 hr to prevent bacterial contamination.

    N NCLEX® Connection: Basic Care and Comfort, Nutrition and Oral Hydration

6. *Using the ATI Active Learning Template: Basic Concept*

   A. Related Content
      - Gastrointestinal disturbance
         ○ Increase the amount of free fluid if constipated.
         ○ Consider a change to formula with enriched fiber if constipated.
         ○ Decrease the flow rate if cramping occurs.
         ○ Give the formula at room temperature.
      - Feeding tube obstruction
         ○ Flush the tubing with 20 to 30 mL of warm water every 4 hr.
         ○ Flush before and after feedings and medication.
         ○ Use a piston syringe with 50 mL of warm water to unclog the tubing.
         ○ Only use carbonated beverage if warm water does not open the tubing.
      - Food poisoning
         ○ Wash hands before handling the formula or equipment.
         ○ Clean tops of formula containers.
         ○ Cover, label, and refrigerate formula up to 24 hr.
         ○ Replace the feeding bag and administration tubing every 24 hr.

   Ⓝ NCLEX® Connection: Reduction of Risk Potential, Potential for Complications of Diagnostic Tests/
   Treatments/Procedures

chapter 10

Overview

- Parenteral nutrition (PN) is used when a client's gastrointestinal tract is not functioning, or when a client cannot physically or psychologically consume sufficient nutrients orally or enterally.

- Based upon the client's nutritional needs and anticipated duration of therapy, PN can be given as either total parenteral nutrition (TPN) or peripheral parenteral nutrition (PPN).

  ○ TPN provides a nutritionally complete solution. It can be used when caloric needs are very high, when the anticipated duration of therapy is greater than 7 days, or when the solution to be administered is hypertonic (composed of greater than 10% dextrose). It can only be administered in a central vein.

  ○ PPN can provide a nutritionally complete solution. However, it is administered into a peripheral vein, resulting in a limited nutritional value. It is indicated for clients who require short-term nutritional support with fewer calories per day. The solution must be isotonic and contain no more than 10% dextrose and 5% amino acids.

Components of Parenteral Nutrition Solutions

- PN includes amino acids, dextrose, electrolytes, vitamins, and trace elements in sterile water.

- Carbohydrate or dextrose solutions are available in concentrations of 5% for PPN and up to 70% for TPN.

  ○ A higher concentration of dextrose is often prescribed for a client on fluid restrictions.

  ○ A lower-dextrose concentration may be used to help control hyperglycemia.

- Electrolytes, vitamins, and trace elements are essential for normal body functions. The amounts added are dependent upon the client's blood chemistry values, and physical assessment findings are used to determine the quantity of electrolytes. Additional vitamin K may be added to the PN solution.

- Lipids (fats) are available in concentrations of 10%, 20%, and 30%. Lipids are a significant source of calories and are used to correct or prevent essential fatty acid deficiency.

  ○ Lipid emulsions can be added to the PN solution, administered piggyback, or given intermittently.

  ○ IV lipids are contraindicated for clients who have hyperlipidemia, severe hepatic disease, or an allergy to soybean oil, eggs, or safflower oil.

  ○ Lipid emulsion provides the needed calories when dextrose concentration must be reduced due to fluid restrictions.

  ○ Lipid emulsion provides the calories without increasing the osmolality of the PN solution.

- Protein is provided as a mixture of essential and nonessential amino acids and is available in concentrations of 3% to 5%.

  ○ Protein should provide 3.5% to 20% of the total concentration of the PN solution.

  ○ The client's estimated requirements and liver and kidney function determine the amount of protein provided.

- Two medications, insulin and heparin, may be added to the PN solution by pharmacy services. Insulin may be added to reduce the potential for hyperglycemia, and heparin may be added to prevent fibrin buildup on the catheter tip. Administering any IV medication through a PN IV line or port is contraindicated.

Indications

- Diagnoses

  ○ TPN is commonly used in clients undergoing treatment for cancer, bowel disorders, and those suffering from trauma or extensive burns, as these conditions are associated with high caloric requirements.

  ○ PPN may be used when central venous access is not available, or for transition from TPN to enteral or oral intake.

Desired Therapeutic Outcomes

- Evidence supporting the effectiveness of PN includes:

  ○ Daily weight gain of up to 1 kg/day.

  ○ Increases in albumin level (expected reference range of 3.5 to 5.0 g/dL) and in prealbumin level (expected reference range of 23 to 43 mg/dL).

Nursing Actions

- Preparation of the Client

  ○ Prior to initiating PN, nurses should review the client's weight, BMI, nutritional status, diagnosis, and current laboratory data. This may include CBC, serum chemistry profile, PT/aPTT, iron, total iron-binding capacity, lipid profile, liver function tests, electrolyte panel, BUN, prealbumin and albumin level, creatinine, blood glucose, and platelet count.

  ○ Assess the client's educational needs.

  ○ An electronic infusion device should be used to prevent the accidental overload of a solution.

  ○ A micron filter on the IV tubing is required when administering PN solution. This filter is not added to the IV tubing when administering a lipid emulsion. Follow facility guidelines when administering all PN solutions.

- Ongoing Care
  - Nursing care is focused on preventing complications through consistent monitoring. Specific monitoring guidelines vary among health care facilities.
    - Ongoing assessment parameters include I&O, daily weights, vital signs, pertinent laboratory values (e.g., serum electrolytes, blood glucose), and ongoing evaluation of the client's underlying condition. This data is used to determine the client's response to therapy and the formulation of the solution to prevent nutrient deficiencies or toxicities.
    - Monitor serum and urine glucose as prescribed and per facility guidelines. Sliding scale insulin may be prescribed to intervene for hyperglycemia, or regular insulin may be added to the PN solution.
    - Flow rate should be monitored carefully.
      - Failure to provide optimal nutritional intake is the result of solutions administered too slowly.
      - Hyperosmolar diuresis can result from an infusion that is too rapid, and can lead to dehydration, hypovolemic shock, seizures, coma, and death.
      - To avoid hypoglycemia, an IV of dextrose 10% to 20% in water is administered if the PN solution is unavailable.
      - Hyperglycemia, hyperosmolar diuresis, and fluid overload may occur if the PN solution is increased when available. Do not attempt to increase the rate of the PN solution to "catch up."

    - Monitor for "cracking" of TPN solution. This occurs if the calcium or phosphorous content is high or if poor-salt albumin is added. A "cracked" TPN solution has an oily appearance or a layer of fat on top of the solution and should not be used.
  - Strict aseptic techniques are maintained to reduce the risk of infection. The high dextrose content of PN contributes to bacterial growth.
  - Use sterile technique when changing central line dressing and tubing. The bag and tubing should be changed every 24 hr or per facility protocol.

 View Video: Total Parenteral Nutrition

- Interventions
  - PN should be discontinued as soon as possible to avoid potential complications, but not until the client's enteral or oral intake can provide 60% or more of estimated caloric requirements.
    - Discontinuation should be done gradually to avoid rebound hypoglycemia.
  - Education for clients and family regarding TPN at home begins with a psychosocial assessment to determine coping and readiness, and then should include aseptic preparation and administration techniques, blood glucose monitoring, and criteria to evaluate for the presence of infection and complications.

Complications

- Infection and sepsis are evidenced by a fever or elevated WBC count. Infection can result from contamination of the catheter during insertion, contaminated solution, or a long-term indwelling catheter.

- Metabolic complications include hyperglycemia, hypoglycemia, hyperkalemia, hypophosphatemia, hypocalcemia, hypoalbuminemia, dehydration, and fluid overload (as evidenced by weight gain greater than 1 kg/day and edema).

- Mechanical complications include catheter misplacement, pneumothorax (evidenced by shortness of breath, diminished or absent breath sounds), subclavian artery puncture, catheter embolus, air embolus, thrombosis, obstruction, and bolus infusion.

APPLICATION EXERCISES

1. A nurse is planning care for a client who has a new prescription for peripheral parenteral nutrition (PPN). Which of the following interventions should the nurse include in the plan of care? (Select all that apply.)

_____ A. Examine trends in weight loss.

_____ B. Review prealbumin finding.

_____ C. Administer an IV solution of 20% dextrose.

_____ D. Add a micron filter to IV tubing.

_____ E. Use an IV infusion pump.

2. A charge nurse is providing information about fat emulsion added to total parenteral nutrition (TPN) to a group of nurses. Which of the following statements by the nurse are appropriate? (Select all that apply.)

_____ A. "Concentration of lipid emulsion can be up to 30%."

_____ B. "Adding lipid emulsion gives the solution a milky appearance."

_____ C. "Check for allergies to soybean oil."

_____ D. "Lipid emulsion prevents essential fatty acid deficiency."

_____ E. "Lipids provide calories by increasing the osmolality of the PN solution."

3. A charge nurse is teaching a group of nurses about medication compatibility with TPN. Which of the following statements by the nurse is appropriate?

A. "Use the Y-port on the TPN IV tubing to administer antibiotics."

B. "Regular insulin may be added to the TPN solution."

C. "Administer heparin through a port on the TPN tubing."

D. "Administer vitamin K IV bolus via a Y-port on the TPN tubing."

4. A nurse is preparing to administer lipid emulsion and notes a layer of fat floating in the IV solution bag. Which of the following is an appropriate action by the nurse?

A. Shake the bag to mix the fat.

B. Turn the bag upside down one time.

C. Return the bag to the pharmacy.

D. Administer the bag of solution.

5. A nurse is caring for a client who is receiving TPN, but the next bag of solution is not available for administration at this time. Which of the following is an appropriate action by the nurse?

    A. Administer 20% dextrose in water IV until the next bag is available.

    B. Slow the infusion rate of the current bag until the solution is available.

    C. Monitor for hyperglycemia.

    D. Monitor for hyperosmolar diuresis.

6. A nurse is teaching a client about complications that can occur when receiving total parenteral nutrition (TPN). What should be included in the teaching? Use the ATI Active Learning Template: Basic Concept to complete this item to include the following:

    A. Related Content:
- Identify three complications of TPN.
- Describe two nursing intervention related to each complication.

APPLICATION EXERCISES KEY

1. A. **CORRECT:** Examining trends in weight loss will help to evaluate the outcome of PPN.

    B. **CORRECT:** Reviewing the prealbumin finding will determine nutritional deficiency over a short period of time.

    C. INCORRECT: An IV solution of 20% dextrose is administered only as total parenteral nutrition (TPN) using a central vein.

    D. **CORRECT:** A micron filter is always used when infusing PN solution.

    E. **CORRECT:** An IV infusion pump is always used to regulate the flow and provide accurate delivery of the PN solution.

    Ⓝ NCLEX® Connection: Pharmacological and Parenteral Therapies, Total Parenteral Nutrition (TPN)

2. A. **CORRECT:** Lipid emulsion is available in 10%, 20%, and 30% concentrations depending upon the carbohydrate and caloric needs for clients.

    B. **CORRECT:** The lipid emulsion is formulated from safflower or soybean oils and egg phospholipid, making the solution appear milky.

    C. **CORRECT:** Lipid emulsion is formulated from safflower or soybean oil and egg phospholipid. The nurse should check for allergies to these ingredients.

    D. **CORRECT:** Lipid emulsion is used for additional calories as concentrated energy and to prevent essential fatty acid deficiency.

    E. INCORRECT: Lipids provide the calories needed without increasing osmolality of the PN solution.

    Ⓝ NCLEX® Connection: Pharmacological and Parenteral Therapies, Total Parenteral Nutrition (TPN)

3. A. INCORRECT: Administering any IV medication through a Y-port on the TPN line is contraindicated.

    B. **CORRECT:** Regular insulin may be added to the TPN solution to decrease hyperglycemia.

    C. INCORRECT: Heparin may be added to the TPN solution to decrease clot formation in the cannula, but it is not injected directly into a port on the TPN tubing.

    D. INCORRECT: Vitamin K can be added to the TPN solution, but it should not be administered IV bolus through the TPN IV line.

    Ⓝ NCLEX® Connection: Pharmacological and Parenteral Therapies, Total Parenteral Nutrition (TPN)

4. A. INCORRECT: Shaking the bag is not an appropriate action because "cracking" of the solution has occurred and it should not be administered.

    B. INCORRECT: Turning the solution upside down does not resolve the problem because "cracking" of the TPN has occurred and it should not be administered.

    C. **CORRECT:** Returning the solution to the pharmacy is an appropriate action by the nurse because "cracking" of the solution has occurred and it should not be administered.

    D. INCORRECT: Administering the solution is not an appropriate nursing action because "cracking" of the solution has occurred.

    Ⓝ NCLEX® Connection: Pharmacological and Parenteral Therapies, Total Parenteral Nutrition (TPN)

5. A. **CORRECT:** Administering 20% dextrose in water IV until the TPN solution is available will avoid hypoglycemia.

    B. INCORRECT: Decreasing the rate of the TPN solution is not an appropriate action because the decreased rate may cause hypoglycemia.

    C. INCORRECT: The client should be monitored for hypoglycemia when the TPN solution is not infusing and if dextrose is not administered.

    D. INCORRECT: The nurse should monitor the client for hyperosmolar diuresis when the TPN solution has infused too fast, this is not an appropriate action at this time.

    Ⓝ NCLEX® Connection: Pharmacological and Parenteral Therapies, Total Parenteral Nutrition (TPN)

6. *Using the ATI Active Learning Template: Basic Concept*

    A. Related Content
    - Infection and sepsis
      - Monitor for manifestations of fever, chills, increased WBCs, and redness around catheter insertion site.
    - Hyperglycemia
      - Administer sliding scale insulin or plan for insulin to be added to the TPN solution.
      - Monitor blood glucose.
    - Hypoglycemia
      - Inform the provider and plan to give additional dextrose.
      - Monitor frequent blood glucose.
    - Weight gain greater than 1 kg/day
      - Inform the provider and anticipate a decrease in the concentration, rate of administration or volume of lipid emulsion.
      - Monitor the client's intake of oral nutrients.

    Ⓝ NCLEX® Connection: Pharmacological and Parenteral Therapies, Total Parenteral Nutrition (TPN)

UNIT 3   Alterations in Nutrition

CHAPTERS

› Barriers to Adequate Nutrition
› Cardiovascular and Hematologic Disorders
› Gastrointestinal Disorders
› Renal Disorders
› Diabetes Mellitus
› Cancer and Immunosuppression Disorders

NCLEX® CONNECTIONS

When reviewing the chapters in this unit, keep in mind the relevant sections of the NCLEX® outline, in particular:

Client Needs: Health Promotion and Maintenance	Client Needs: Basic Care and Comfort	Client Needs: Physiological Adaptation
› Relevant topics/tasks include: » Health Promotion/Disease Prevention › Identify risk factors for disease/illness. » Health Screening › Identify risk factors linked to ethnicity. » High-Risk Behaviors › Assist the client to identify behaviors/risks that may impact health.	› Relevant topics/tasks include: » Nutrition and Oral Hydration › Provide nutritional supplements as needed. › Manage the client who has an alteration in nutritional intake. › Evaluate the impact of disease/illness on the nutritional status of the client.	› Relevant topics/tasks include: » Alterations in Body Systems › Assess the adaptation of the client to health alteration, illness, and/or disease. › Educate the client about managing health problems. › Implement interventions to address side/adverse effects of radiation therapy.

chapter 11

Overview

- Many individuals have difficulty consuming a nutritional or prescribed diet due to factors that create a barrier.

- Medical, psychological, and social factors can all create nutritional barriers.

- It is important for nurses to recognize these factors as nutritional education will be ineffective if a client lacks the necessary resources to follow through on recommendations.

- Barriers to client nutrition that nurses commonly have to acknowledge are:

  - Poor dentition, dental caries, or poorly fitting dentures

  - Low socioeconomic status and lack of access

  - Cognitive disorders

  - Altered sensory perception

  - Impairment in swallowing

  - Mechanical fixation of the jaw

  - Lack of knowledge and misinformation about nutrition

Nutritional Barriers and Nursing Interventions

- Poor Dentition, Dental Caries, or Poorly Fitting Dentures

  - Poor dentition is a potential problem for clients across the lifespan.

    - Children who do not have access to dental care or tools (toothbrush, toothpaste) may have caries that impair the ability to chew.

    - Adults who have lost teeth or have teeth that need removal or repair will have an impaired ability to chew.

    - After an adult has teeth removed, it may be difficult to adjust to dentures.

  - Nursing Care

    - School screenings can help identify children who need dental attention, and can facilitate the referral process.

    - Provide children with information about healthy snacks that are low in sugar content.

    - Advise children and adults to limit consumption of processed carbohydrates, which can stick to teeth and increase the risk for dental caries.

    - Encourage children and adults to use a fluoridated tooth paste and have fluoride applied to their teeth.

- Adults who are admitted to acute or long-term care facilities should have a dental inspection done by a nurse to identify issues that may impact the ability to properly eat.

- If a barrier is found to exist, consult a dietician so the proper diet is prescribed and nutritional supplements are added as necessary.

- Low Socioeconomic Status and Lack of Access

  - The lack of money to purchase healthy foods or foods required for a special diet can be a barrier to maintaining a proper diet.

    - Nutritious foods (fresh fruit, vegetables) tend to be more expensive than canned and boxed foods.

    - Canned and boxed foods are usually high in calories and salt, and often contain a higher fat and simple carbohydrate content. These are poor choices for clients on calorie- or sodium-restricted diets.

    - The lack of money to purchase necessary food can lead to malnutrition or obesity if canned and boxed foods are selected.

    - The lack of transportation to grocery stores is a barrier if the client does not have a car or is not licensed to drive.

  - Nursing Care

    - Refer the client to a dietician who can discuss food options and substitutions that are appropriate.

    - Frozen fruits and vegetables may be an affordable option, and are maintained longer in the freezer.

    - Educate clients on how to read food labels to be aware of nutritional, caloric, and sodium values of the food they are consuming.

    - Contact social services regarding the availability of food or meal delivery to the client's home. Investigate the availability of a nutrition program for older adults that provide a noon meal for a localized community.

- Cognitive Disorders

  - Cognitive disorders (dementia, Alzheimer's disease [AD]) may have a significant impact on nutritional status.

    - Clients who have dementia or AD may experience impairments in memory and judgment, making shopping and food selection difficult.

    - As dementia and AD progress, clients may refuse to eat or choose a small selection of food that may not provide adequate nutrition.

  - Nursing Care

    - If the client lives independently, encourage shopping with a friend or family member, and to follow a shopping list.

    - Monitor for vitamin and mineral deficits, and evaluate the need for nutritional supplements.

    - Contact social services regarding the availability of food or meal delivery to the client's home.

    - If the client lives in a care facility, provide a menu with minimal but nutritious options.

    - Serve meals at the same time and in the same location surrounded by the same residents. Keep environmental distractions to a minimum.

    - Provide snacks in between meals if meal time intake is inadequate.

    - Cut food into small pieces if the client does has difficulty chewing food. Remind the client to chew and then swallow. Lightly stroking the chin and throat may help promote swallowing.

- Altered Sensory Perception
  - ○ Clients who have an alteration in vision, smell, or taste may find it difficult to feed themselves or may find food unpalatable.
    - Clients who have decreased vision may need assistance shopping for food on a regular basis, and with food preparation.
    - Clients in a health or long-term care facility will need help with tray setup and location of food on the tray.
    - Clients who have an altered sense of smell will have an altered sense of taste.
    - Clients who smoke can have a diminished sense of smell.
    - Clients on chemotherapy and other types of medications can have an unusual taste in their mouth (metallic taste), masking the real taste of food.
    - Clients on chemotherapy can experience nausea and anorexia, resulting in an aversion to food.

  - ○ Nursing Care
    - Encourage the client who has decreased vision to shop with a friend or family member, or have groceries delivered to the house.
    - Contact social services regarding availability of food or meal delivery to the client's home.
    - Recommend to the client who has a food aversion to eat foods that are served cool, as they are typically less aromatic and are less likely to precipitate nausea.
    - Suggest consuming foods that are spicy or tangy to compensate for the decreased sense of taste.
    - Recommend sucking on hard candies, mints, or chewing gum to counteract an unusual taste in the mouth.
    - Instruct the client to avoid ingestion of empty calories. If an increase in calories and fluid is desired, milkshakes, juice, and supplements are good options.

- Impairment in Swallowing
  - ○ Clients who have neurological disorders (Parkinson's disease, cerebral palsy, stroke) or had a surgical procedure done on their mouth, throat, epiglottis, or larynx can have difficulty managing food and swallowing without choking.
    - Clients who have a neurological disorder affecting the muscles in their mouth and throat are at risk for aspiration due to delayed swallowing and/or inadequate mastication.
    - Clients who have a history of oral cancer may have had part of their lip, tongue, and/or soft palate removed. This significantly affects the ability to masticate and coordinate the development of a bolus of food prior to swallowing.
    - Clients who have had their epiglottis completely or partially removed, or part of their larynx removed, have an anatomical structure removed that previously prevented food from entering the trachea. Unless special precautions are taken, the client will easily aspirate food and fluids consumed.

  - ○ Nursing Care
    - Continually monitor clients who are at risk for aspiration during meals, and have suction equipment immediately available.
    - Consult a dietician regarding an appropriate diet for the client (thick liquids, pureed, mechanical soft).

- ▪ Thicken thin fluids with a commercial thickener to the prescribed consistency of a nectar, honey, or pudding.

- ▪ Teach clients who aspirate easily due to surgical alteration of their throat or upper tracheal structures to tuck their chins when swallowing. Arching the tongue in the back of the throat may help close off the trachea.

- • Mechanical Fixation of the Jaw
  - ○ Disorders of the jaw requiring surgery include facial trauma and reconstruction.
    - ▪ After fractured bones are realigned, the client's upper and lower jaw may be wired together.
    - ▪ The jaw may be immobilized for several weeks.
    - ▪ The client may be placed on a liquid diet during this period.
  - ○ Nursing Care
    - ▪ Encourage the intake of fluids
    - ▪ Help the client determine where to insert a straw through the space between the jaws

    - ▪ Work with the dietician to develop a liquid meal plan that includes the necessary nutrients

- • Lack of Knowledge and Misinformation about Nutrition
  - ○ Clients who do not have a good understanding about nutritional needs may be subject to overnutrition, undernutrition, and the ingestion of an inadequate intake of essential nutrients.
    - ▪ Clients may not have basic knowledge about nutrition.
    - ▪ Information about nutrition may be confusing or misleading.
    - ▪ Clients may be drawn to fad diets (which are generally unhealthy) because quick results are promised.
    - ▪ Clients can be misled by false advertising.
  - ○ Nursing Care
    - ▪ Encourage clients to use dietary guidelines available from government and health associations (MyPlate [www.choosemyplate.gov], the American Heart Association).
    - ▪ Assist clients in locating community resources that provide education on nutrition.
    - ▪ Perform an assessment of dietary intake.
    - ▪ Instruct clients on how to read nutrition fact labels.
    - ▪ Provide clients with information on foods that are healthy and portion sizes.
    - ▪ Warn clients that advertisements may be fraudulent.

APPLICATION EXERCISES

1. A nurse is caring for several clients in an extended care facility. Which of the following clients is the highest priority to observe during meals?

    A. A client who has decreased vision

    B. A client who has Parkinson's disease

    C. A client who has poor dentition

    D. A client who has anorexia

2. A nurse is planning care for an older adult client who is receiving treatment for malnutrition. The client is scheduled for discharge to his home where he lives alone. Which of the following actions are appropriate to include in the plan of care? (Select all that apply.)

    _____ A. Consult social services to arrange home meal delivery.

    _____ B. Encourage the client to purchase nonperishable boxed meals.

    _____ C. Advise the client to purchase frozen fruits and vegetables.

    _____ D. Recommend drinking a supplement between meals.

    _____ E. Educate the client on how to read nutrition labels.

3. A nurse is providing teaching for a client who has a new diagnosis of hypertension and a prescription for a low-sodium diet. Which of the following client statements indicates a need for further teaching?

    A. "I should select organic canned vegetables."

    B. "I need to read food labels when grocery shopping."

    C. "I will stop eating frozen dinners for lunch at work."

    D. "I know that deli meats are usually high in sodium."

4. A nurse is caring for a client who is transitioning to an oral diet following a partial laryngectomy. Which of the following actions by the nurse is appropriate?

    A. Request to have the client's oral medications provided in liquid form.

    B. Instruct the client to follow each bite of food with a drink of water.

    C. Encourage the client to tuck the chin when swallowing.

    D. Consult the dietician about providing the client with a thin liquid diet.

5. A nurse is planning care for a client who has mechanical fixation of the jaw following a motorcycle crash. Which of the following actions are appropriate to include in the plan of care? (Select all that apply.)

_____ A. Thicken the client's liquids to honey consistency.

_____ B. Educate the client about the use of a nasogastric tube.

_____ C. Assist the client to use a straw to drink liquids.

_____ D. Ensure that the client receives ground meats.

_____ E. Encourage the client's intake of fluids between meals.

6. A nurse is providing dietary teaching for a client who requests assistance for weight loss. The client states, "I've tried several fad diets but they don't work for me." Use the ATI Active Learning Template: Basic Concept to complete this item to include the following sections:

A. Underlying Principles: Identify the client's barrier to nutrition.

B. Nursing Interventions: Identify at least four interventions to address this client's barrier to nutrition and to promote healthy weight loss.

APPLICATION EXERCISES KEY

1. A. INCORRECT: Observation of a client who has decreased vision may be necessary to evaluate the client's need for assistance. However, this client is not the highest priority to observe during meals.

    B. **CORRECT:** A client who has Parkinson's disease is at risk for aspiration. Due to this safety risk, this client is the highest priority to observe during meals.

    C. INCORRECT: Observation of a client who has poor dentition may be necessary to evaluate the client's need for assistance or a modified diet. However, this client is not the highest priority to observe during meals.

    D. INCORRECT: Observation of a client who has anorexia may be necessary to evaluate the client's intake. However, this client is not the highest priority to observe during meals.

    (N) NCLEX® Connection: Safety and Infection Control, Accident/Error/Injury Prevention

2. A. **CORRECT:** Consulting social services to arrange home meal delivery is an appropriate action to promote adequate nutrition.

    B. INCORRECT: Boxed foods are usually high in calories and salt, and are therefore not an appropriate action to promote adequate nutrition.

    C. **CORRECT:** Advising the client to purchase frozen fruits and vegetables is an appropriate action to promote adequate nutrition.

    D. **CORRECT:** Recommending a supplement between meals is an appropriate action to promote adequate nutrition.

    E. **CORRECT:** Educating the client on how to read food labels is an appropriate action to promote adequate nutrition.

    (N) NCLEX® Connection: Physiological Adaptations, Illness Management

3. A. **CORRECT:** This statement requires further teaching. Canned foods are usually high in sodium and are therefore a poor choice for a client on a sodium-restricted diet.

    B. INCORRECT: Reading food labels provides the client with information about the food's sodium content.

    C. INCORRECT: Frozen dinners are usually high in sodium and are therefore a poor choice for a client on a sodium-restricted diet.

    D. INCORRECT: Deli meats are usually high in sodium and are therefore a poor choice for a client on a sodium-restricted diet.

    (N) NCLEX® Connection: Basic Care and Comfort, Nutrition and Oral Hydration

4. A. INCORRECT: Providing medications in liquid form does not decrease the risk for aspiration.

    B. INCORRECT: Drinking thin liquids, such as water, increases the risk for aspiration.

    C. **CORRECT:** Tucking the chin when swallowing helps to close off the trachea and reduces the risk for aspiration.

    D. INCORRECT: Thick, rather than thin, liquids help reduce the risk for aspiration.

    Ⓝ NCLEX® Connection: Reduction of Risk Potential, Potential for Complications of Diagnostic Tests/ Treatments/Procedures

5. A. INCORRECT: Mechanical fixation of the jaw does not cause dysphagia. Therefore, it is not necessary to thicken the client's liquids.

    B. INCORRECT: Mechanical fixation of the jaw does not indicate the need for a nasogastric tube.

    C. **CORRECT:** Helping the client use a straw is an appropriate action. The nurse should help the client determine where to insert the straw through the space between the jaws.

    D. INCORRECT: Mechanical fixation of the jaw indicates the need for a liquid diet rather than ground meats.

    E. **CORRECT:** The nurse should encourage the intake of fluids for a client who has mechanical fixation of the jaw.

    Ⓝ NCLEX® Connection: Physiological Adaptations, Illness Management

6. *Using the ATI Active Learning Template: Basic Concept*

    A. Underlying Principles
    - The client's barrier to nutrition is lack of knowledge and misinformation about nutrition. This barrier must be acknowledged to promote adequate nutrition.

    B. Nursing Interventions
    - Encourage the client to use dietary guidelines such as MyPlate.
    - Assist the client in locating community resources that provide education and nutrition to support healthy nutrition and weight loss.
    - Advise the clients that fad diets are generally unhealthy and often include false advertising.
    - Perform an assessment of dietary intake.
    - Encourage the client to keep a journal of dietary intake.
    - Provide the client with information on healthy foods and portion sizes.

    Ⓝ NCLEX® Connection: Health Promotion and Maintenance, Health Promotion/Disease Prevention

chapter 12

Overview

- Nurses must have an awareness of nutritional needs for clients who have cardiovascular and hematologic disorders. It is important to explore dietary needs with the client and recommend modifications related to the disease process. Understanding the role of primary and secondary prevention is essential to successful treatment.
- Specific nutritional considerations are covered in this chapter for:
  - Coronary heart disease
  - Hypertension
  - Heart failure
  - Myocardial infarction
  - Anemia
  - Metabolic syndrome
- Cardiovascular diseases are the leading cause of death in the United States. Coronary heart disease (CHD) is the single leading cause of death.

Assessment/Data Collection

- Coronary Heart Disease
  - Hypercholesterolemia is a major risk factor for developing CHD. CHD is caused by atherosclerosis, a process of damage and cholesterol deposits on the blood vessels of the heart.
    - High density lipoprotein (HDL) cholesterol is "good" cholesterol because it removes cholesterol from the serum and takes it to the liver. The expected reference range HDL for females is 35 to 80 mg/dL, and 35 to 65 mg/dL for males.
    - Low density lipoprotein (LDL) cholesterol is "bad" cholesterol because it transports cholesterol out of the liver and into the circulatory system, where it can form plaques on the coronary artery walls. The expected reference range for LDL is less than 130 mg/dL.

- Evidence has demonstrated that a diet high in cholesterol and saturated fats greatly increases the risk of developing heart disease.
- Anemia
  - Iron Deficiency Anemia
    - Manifestations
      - Fatigue
      - Lethargy
      - Pallor of nail beds
      - Intolerance to cold
    - Children with low iron intake can experience short attention spans and display poor intellectual performance before anemia begins.

- ○ Macrocytic Anemia
  - ▪ Manifestations
    - □ Pallor
    - □ Weakness
    - □ Palpitations
    - □ Dyspnea
    - □ Fatigue
- ○ Vitamin B$_{12}$ Deficiency Anemia
  - ▪ Gastrointestinal Findings
    - □ Glossitis (inflamed tongue)
    - □ Anorexia
    - □ Indigestion
    - □ Weight loss
    - □ Frequent diarrhea and/or constipation
  - ▪ Neurological Findings
    - □ Paresthesia (numbness) of hands and feet
    - □ Decreased proprioception (sense of body position)
    - □ Poor muscle coordination
    - □ Increasing irritability
    - □ Delirium
- ○ Folic Acid Deficiency Anemia
  - ▪ Manifestations include mental confusion, fainting, fatigue, and gastrointestinal distress.
  - ▪ Findings of folic acid deficiency anemia mimic those for vitamin B$_{12}$ deficiency anemia except for the neurological manifestations.
- • Metabolic Syndrome
  - ○ The presence of three of the five following risk factors:
  - ○ Abdominal obesity
    - ▪ Men: greater than 40-inch waist
    - ▪ Women: greater than 35-inch waist
  - ○ Triglycerides greater than 150 mg/dL
  - ○ Low HDL
    - ▪ Men: less than 40 mg/dL
    - ▪ Women: less than 50 mg/dL
  - ○ Increased blood pressure
    - ▪ Systolic greater than or equal to 130 mm/Hg
    - ▪ Diastolic greater than or equal to 85 mm/Hg
  - ○ Fasting blood glucose greater than or equal to 110 mg/dL

Nutritional Guidelines and Nursing Interventions

- Coronary Heart Disease
  - Preventative Nutrition
    - Consuming a low-fat, low-cholesterol diet can reduce the risk of developing CHD. The Therapeutic Lifestyle Change (TLC) diet is designed to be a user-friendly eating guide to encourage dietary changes.
    - Daily cholesterol intake should be less than 200 mg.
    - Conservative use of red wine may reduce the risk of developing CHD.
    - Increasing fiber and carbohydrate intake, avoiding saturated fat, and decreasing red meat consumption can decrease the risk for developing CHD.
    - Increased intake of omega-3 fatty acids found in fish, flaxseed, soy beans, canola, and walnuts reduces the risk of coronary artery disease.
    - Homocysteine is an amino acid. Elevated homocysteine levels can increase the risk of developing CHD. Deficiencies in folate and vitamins B_6 and B_{12} increase homocysteine levels.
  - Therapeutic Nutrition
    - Secondary prevention efforts for CHD are focused on lifestyle changes that lower LDL. These include a diet low in cholesterol and saturated fats, a diet high in fiber, exercise and weight management, and smoking cessation.
    - Daily cholesterol intake should be less than 200 mg/day. Saturated fat should be limited to less than 7% of daily caloric intake.
    - To lower cholesterol and saturated fats, instruct the client to:
      - Trim visible fat from meats.
      - Limit red meats and choose lean meats (turkey, chicken).
      - Remove the skin from meats.
      - Broil, bake, grill, or steam foods. Avoid frying foods.
      - Use low-fat or nonfat milk, cheese, and yogurt.
      - Use spices in place of butter or salt to season foods.
      - Avoid trans fat as it increases LDL. Partially hydrogenated products contain trans fat.
      - Read labels.
    - Encourage the client to consume a high-fiber diet. Soluble fiber lowers LDL.
      - Oats, beans, fruits, vegetables, whole grains, barley, and flaxseed are good sources of fiber.
    - Encourage the client to exercise.
      - Instruct the client regarding practical methods for increasing physical activity. (Encourage the client to take the stairs rather than the elevator.)
      - Provide the client with references for local exercise facilities.
    - Instruct the client to stop all use of tobacco products.
    - The recommended lifestyle changes represent a significant change for many clients.
      - Provide support to the client and family.
      - Encourage the client's family to participate in the changes to ease the transition for the client.

- □ Explain why the diet is important.
- □ Aid the client in developing a diet that is complementary to personal food preferences and lifestyle. A food diary may be helpful.
- □ Instruct the client that occasional deviations from the diet are reasonable.

- Hypertension
  - ○ Hypertension is a significant risk factor for developing CHD, myocardial infarction, and stroke.
  - ○ Hypertension is a sustained elevation in blood pressure greater than or equal to 140/90 mm/Hg.
  - ○ Therapeutic Nutrition
    - ▪ The Dietary Approaches to Stopping Hypertension (DASH) diet is a low-sodium, high-potassium, high-calcium diet that has proven to lower blood pressure (systolic and diastolic) and cholesterol.
      - □ Decrease sodium intake (a daily intake of less than 2,400 mg is recommended).
      - □ Foods high in sodium include canned soups and sauces, potato chips, pretzels, smoked meats, seasonings, and processed foods.
      - □ Include low-fat dairy products to promote calcium intake.
      - □ Include fruits and vegetables rich in potassium (apricots, bananas, tomatoes, potatoes).
    - ▪ Limit alcohol intake.
    - ▪ Encourage the client to read labels and educate the client about appropriate food choices.
    - ▪ Other lifestyle changes include exercising, weight loss, and smoking cessation.

- Heart Failure
  - ○ Heart failure is characterized by the inability of the heart to maintain adequate blood flow throughout the circulatory system. It results in excess sodium and fluid retention, and edema.
  - ○ Therapeutic Nutrition
    - ▪ Reduce sodium intake to 2,000 mg/day or less.
    - ▪ Monitor (and possibly restrict to 1.5 L/day) fluid intake.

- Myocardial Infarction (MI)
  - ○ An MI occurs when there is an inadequate supply of oxygen to the myocardium. Frequently an MI occurs because of atherosclerosis.
  - ○ After an MI, it is necessary to reduce the myocardial oxygen demands related to metabolic activity.
  - ○ Therapeutic Nutrition
    - ▪ A liquid diet is best for the first 24 hr after the infarction.
    - ▪ Caffeine should be avoided because it stimulates the heart and increases heart rate.
    - ▪ Small, frequent meals are indicated.
    - ▪ Counsel the client about recommendations for a heart-healthy diet.

- Anemia
  - ○ Anemia results from either a reduction in the number of red blood cells (RBCs) or in hemoglobin, the oxygen-carrying component of blood. Anemia can result from a decrease in RBC production, an increase in RBC destruction, or a loss of blood.
    - ▪ The body requires iron, vitamin B_{12}, and folic acid to produce red blood cells.
    - ▪ Iron deficiency anemia is the most common nutritional disorder in the world. It affects approximately 10% of the U.S. population, especially older infants, toddlers, adolescent girls, and pregnant women.

- From childhood until adolescence, iron intake tends to be marginal.
- Pernicious anemia is the most common form of vitamin B_{12} deficiency. It is caused by lack of intrinsic factor, a protein that helps the body absorb vitamin B_{12}. Risk factors include gastric surgery, gastric cancer, *Helicobacter pylori*, and age greater than 50. Clients who have pernicious anemia require vitamin B_{12} injections.

○ Iron deficiency anemia can result from poor intestinal absorption, blood loss, and inadequate consumption.

- Sources of iron
  □ Meat
  □ Fish
  □ Poultry
  □ Tofu
  □ Dried peas and beans
  □ Whole grains
  □ Dried fruit
- Iron-fortified foods
  □ Infant formula (acceptable alternative or supplement to breastfeeding)
  □ Infant cereal (usually the first food introduced to infants)
  □ Ready-to-eat cereals

- Vitamin C facilitates the absorption of iron (promote consumption).
- Caution: Medicinal iron overdose is the leading cause of accidental poisoning in small children and can lead to acute iron toxicity.

○ Vitamin B_{12} deficiency anemia results from a failure to absorb vitamin B_{12} (pernicious anemia) or inadequate intake.

- Natural sources of vitamin B_{12}
  □ Fish
  □ Meat
  □ Poultry
  □ Eggs
  □ Milk
- People over the age of 50 are urged to consume most of their vitamin B_{12} requirement from supplements or fortified food.
- Vegans need supplemental B_{12}.

○ Folic acid deficiency anemia is caused by poor nutrition, malabsorption (Crohn's disease), and drug use.

- Folic acid sources
  □ Green leafy vegetables
  □ Dried peas and beans
  □ Seeds
  □ Orange juice
  □ Cereals and breads fortified with folic acid
- If the client is unable to obtain an adequate supply of folic acid, supplementation may be necessary.

APPLICATION EXERCISES

1. A nurse is teaching a client about high-fiber foods that can assist in lowering LDL. Which of the following foods should be included in the teaching? (Select all that apply.)

_____ A. Beans

_____ B. Cheese

_____ C. Whole grains

_____ D. Broccoli

_____ E. Yogurt

2. A nurse is teaching a client about dietary recommendations to lower high blood pressure. Which of the following statements by the client indicates the teaching is effective?

A. "My daily sodium consumption should be 3,000 mg."

B. "I should consume foods low in potassium."

C. "My limit is three cigarettes a day."

D. "I should consume low-fat dairy products."

3. A community health nurse is assessing a client who reports numbness of the hands and feet for the past 2 weeks. This finding is associated with which of the following nutritional deficiencies?

A. Folic acid

B. Potassium

C. Vitamin B_{12}

D. Iron

4. A nurse is reviewing a client health record that includes a report of weight gain in the abdomen and laboratory findings of elevated blood glucose and elevated triglycerides. The client is exhibiting clinical manifestations of

A. anemia.

B. metabolic syndrome.

C. heart failure.

D. hypertension.

5. A nurse is providing teaching to a client who has vitamin B_{12} deficiency. Which of the following foods should the nurse instruct the client to consume? (Select all that apply.)

_____ A. Meat

_____ B. Flaxseed

_____ C. Beans

_____ D. Eggs

_____ E. Milk

6. A nurse is providing teaching to a client who has hypertension. What should be included in the teaching? Use the ATI Active Learning Template: Systems Disorder to complete this item to include the following sections:

A. Description of Disorder/Disease Process

B. Client Education: Describe four nutrition teaching points to include a description of the Dietary Approaches to Stopping Hypertension (DASH) diet.

APPLICATION EXERCISES KEY

1. A. **CORRECT:** Beans are a food source high in fiber and should be included in the teaching.

    B. INCORRECT: Cheese is a food source high in calcium and should not be included in the teaching.

    C. **CORRECT:** Whole grains are a food source high in fiber and should be included in the teaching.

    D. **CORRECT:** Broccoli is a food source high in fiber and should be included in the teaching.

    E. INCORRECT: Yogurt is a food source high in calcium and should not be included in the teaching.

    Ⓝ NCLEX® Connection: Basic Care and Comfort, Nutrition and Oral Hydration

2. A. INCORRECT: Daily sodium consumption should be 2,400 mg or less. This assists with lowering systolic and diastolic blood pressures as well as cholesterol.

    B. INCORRECT: Foods high in potassium should be encouraged. This assists with lowering systolic and diastolic blood pressures as well as cholesterol.

    C. INCORRECT: Smoking cessation should be encouraged. Smoking can increase blood pressure and should be avoided.

    D. **CORRECT:** Low-fat dairy products should be encouraged. They promote calcium intake and assist with lowering systolic and diastolic blood pressures as well as cholesterol.

    Ⓝ NCLEX® Connection: Basic Care and Comfort, Nutrition and Oral Hydration

3. A. INCORRECT: Mental confusion, fatigue, fainting, and gastrointestinal distress are clinical manifestations associated with folic acid deficiency.

    B. INCORRECT: Irritability, decreased respirations, muscle weakness, and gastrointestinal distress are clinical manifestations associated with hypokalemia.

    C. **CORRECT:** Numbness of the hands and feet are clinical manifestations associated with vitamin B_{12} deficiency.

    D. INCORRECT: Fatigue, lethargy, pallor of nail beds, and intolerance to cold are clinical manifestations associated with iron deficiency anemia.

    Ⓝ NCLEX® Connection: Basic Care and Comfort, Nutrition and Oral Hydration

4.   A. INCORRECT: Fatigue, lethargy, pallor of nail beds, and intolerance to cold are clinical manifestations associated with anemia.

     B. **CORRECT:** Weight gain in the abdomen, elevated blood glucose, and elevated triglycerides are clinical manifestations associated with metabolic syndrome.

     C. INCORRECT: Shortness of breath, fluid retention, and fatigue are clinical manifestations associated with heart failure.

     D. INCORRECT: Headaches, tiredness, and dizziness are clinical manifestations associated with hypertension.

     N NCLEX® Connection: Basic Care and Comfort, Nutrition and Oral Hydration

5.   A. **CORRECT:** Meat is a food source that is high in vitamin B_{12}.

     B. INCORRECT: Flaxseed is a good source of fiber.

     C. INCORRECT: Beans are a good source of folic acid.

     D. **CORRECT:** Eggs are a food source that is high in vitamin B_{12}.

     E. **CORRECT:** Milk is a food source that is high in vitamin B_{12}.

     N NCLEX® Connection: Basic Care and Comfort, Nutrition and Oral Hydration

6.   *Using the ATI Active Learning Template: Systems Disorder*

     A. Description of Disorder/Disease Process
         • Hypertension is a sustained elevation in blood pressure greater than or equal to 140/90 mm Hg.

     B. Client Education
         • The Dietary Approaches to Stopping Hypertension (DASH) diet is a low-sodium, high-potassium, high-calcium diet that has proven to lower blood pressure and cholesterol.
           ○ Lower sodium intake (a daily intake of less than 2,400 mg is recommended).
             ▪ Foods high in sodium include canned soups and sauces, potato chips, pretzels, smoked meats, seasonings, and processed foods.
           ○ Include low-fat dairy products to promote calcium intake.
           ○ Include fruits and vegetables rich in potassium (apricots, bananas, tomatoes, potatoes).
           ○ Limit alcohol intake.

     N NCLEX® Connection: Physiological Adaptations, Illness Management

chapter 13

Overview

- Nurses must gain an awareness of nutritional needs for clients who have gastrointestinal disorders. It is important to explore dietary needs with the client and recommend modifications in relationship to the disease process. Understanding the role of primary and secondary prevention is essential to successful treatment.

- Specific nutrition considerations covered in this chapter
  - Nausea and vomiting
  - Anorexia
  - Constipation
  - Diarrhea
  - Dysphagia
  - Dumping syndrome
  - Gastroesophageal reflux disease
  - Gastritis
  - Peptic ulcer disease
  - Lactose intolerance
  - Ileostomies and colostomies
  - Diverticulosis and diverticulitis
  - Inflammatory bowel disease
  - Cholecystitis
  - Pancreatitis
  - Liver disease
  - Celiac disease

- Nutrition therapy for gastrointestinal disorders is generally aimed at minimizing or preventing symptoms. In some conditions, such as celiac disease, nutrition is the only treatment.

- For some gastrointestinal disorders, nutrition therapy is the foundation of treatment.

Assessment/Data Collection

- Assess if the client is experiencing any of the following:
  - Difficulty chewing or swallowing, nausea or vomiting, or diarrhea
  - Bloating, excessive flatus, occult blood, steatorrhea, abdominal pain and/or cramping, abdominal distention, pale, sticky bowel movements
  - Changes in weight, eating patterns, or bowel habits
- Assess if the client uses:
  - Tobacco
  - Alcohol
  - Caffeine
  - Over-the-counter medications to treat gastrointestinal conditions (many can have GI complications or be contradicted with GI conditions)
  - Nutritional supplements
  - Herbal supplements for GI conditions or other problems (some clients do not consider them to be medications, so they do not mention them to the provider)

Nutritional Guidelines and Nursing Interventions

- General Gastrointestinal Considerations
  - Monitor gastrointestinal parameters.
    - Weight and weight changes
    - Laboratory values
    - Bowel sounds
    - Elimination patterns
    - I&O
  - Low-fiber diets avoid foods that are high in residue content (whole-grain breads and cereals, raw fruits and vegetables).
    - Diets low in fiber reduce the frequency and volume of fecal output and slow transit time of food through the digestive tract. Low fiber in the diet reduces the frequency and volume of fecal output and slows transit time.
    - Low-fiber diets are used short-term for clients who have diarrhea or malabsorption syndromes.
  - High-fiber diets focus on foods containing more than 5 g of fiber per serving. A diet high in fiber helps:
    - Increase stool bulk.
    - Stimulate peristalsis.
    - Prevent constipation.
    - Protect against colon cancer.

- Nausea and Vomiting
  - ○ Potential causes of nausea and vomiting include decreased gastric acid secretion; decreased gastrointestinal motility; allergy to food(s); bacterial or viral infection; increased intracranial pressure; liver, pancreatic, and gall bladder disorders; or adverse effects of some medications.
  - ○ The underlying cause of nausea and vomiting should be investigated. Assessing the appearance of the emesis will aid in diagnosis and treatment (i.e., coffee-ground emesis indicates the presence of blood; pale green indicates bile).
  - ○ Once manifestations subside, begin with clear liquids followed by full liquids, and advance the diet as tolerated.
  - ○ Easy-to-digest, low-fat carbohydrate foods (crackers, toast, oatmeal, pretzels, plain bread, bland fruit) are usually well-tolerated.
  - ○ Other interventions include:
    - Clients should avoid liquids with meals as they promote a feeling of fullness.
    - Promote good oral hygiene with toothbrushing, mouth swabs, mouthwash, and ice chips.
    - Elevate the head of the bed.
    - Discourage hot and spicy foods.
    - Serve foods at room temperature or chilled.
    - Avoid high-fat foods if they contribute to nausea because they are difficult to digest.
- Anorexia
  - ○ Anorexia is defined as a lack of appetite. It is a common finding for numerous physical conditions and is an adverse effect of certain medications. It is not the same as anorexia nervosa.
  - ○ Anorexia can lead to decreased nutritional intake and subsequent protein and calorie deficits.
  - ○ Nursing Interventions
    - Decrease stress at meal times.
    - Assess for adverse effects of medications.
    - Administer medications to stimulate appetite.
    - Assess and modify environment for unpleasant odors.
    - Remove items that cause a decrease in appetite (soiled linens, garbage, emesis basins, bedpans, used tissues, clutter).
    - Assess and manage anxiety and depression.
    - Provide small, frequent meals and avoid high-fat foods to help maximize the intake of clients who are anorexic.
    - Provide liquid supplements between meals to improve protein and calorie intake.
    - Ensure that meals appear appealing. Serve larger meals early in the day.
    - Assess for changes in bowel status (increased gastric emptying, constipation, diarrhea).
    - Position to increase gastric motility.
    - Provide mouth care before and after meals.

- Constipation
  - Clients who have constipation have difficult or infrequent passage of stools, which may be hard and dry.
  - Causes include irregular bowel habits, psychogenic factors, inactivity, chronic laxative use or abuse, obstruction, medications, GI disorders such as IBS, pregnancy, or secondary to genital/rectal trauma such sexual abuse or child birth, and inadequate consumption of fiber and fluid.
  - Encourage exercise and a diet high in fiber (25 g/day for women and 38 g/day for men), and promote adequate fluid intake to help alleviate symptoms.
  - If caused from medication, a change in the medication may be required.
  - Nursing Interventions
    - Assess onset and duration of past and present elimination patterns, what is normal for the client, activity levels, occupation, dietary intake, and stress levels.
    - Assess past medical and surgical history, medication use (OTC, herbal supplements, laxatives, enemas, and prescriptions), presence of rectal pressure or fullness, and abdominal pain.
    - Encourage client to gradually increase daily intake of fiber.
    - Advise the client that an increase in fiber intake is the preferred treatment for constipation. Chronic use of laxatives should be avoided.
- Diarrhea
  - May cause significant losses of potassium, sodium, and fluid, as well as nutritional complications.
  - Common causes of diarrhea include emotional and physical stress, gastrointestinal disorders, malabsorption disorders, infections, and certain drug therapies.
  - A high-fiber diet may be prescribed, unless it is the fiber that is causing the diarrhea
  - Nutrition therapy varies with the severity and duration of diarrhea. A liberal fluid intake to replace losses is needed.
- Dysphagia
  - Dysphagia is an alteration in the client's ability to swallow.
  - Causes include obstruction, inflammation, and certain neurological disorders.
  - Modifying the texture of foods and the consistency of liquids may enable the client to achieve proper nutrition.
  - Dry mouth can contribute to dysphagia. Evaluate medications being taken.

  - Clients who have dysphagia are at an increased risk of aspiration. Place the client in an upright or high-Fowler's position to facilitate swallowing.
  - Provide oral care prior to eating to enhance the client's sense of taste.
  - Clients who have dysphagia should be referred to a speech therapist for evaluation.
  - Dietary modifications are based on the specific swallowing limitations experienced by the client.
  - Allow adequate time for eating, use adaptive eating devices, and encourage small bites and thorough chewing.
  - Pills should be taken with at least 8 oz of fluid (can be thickened) to prevent medication from remaining in the esophagus.
  - Avoid thin liquids and sticky foods.
  - Nutritional supplements may be indicated if nutritional intake is deemed inadequate.

- Dumping syndrome
  - Normally, the stomach controls the rate in which nutrients enter the small intestine. When a portion of the stomach is surgically removed, the contents of the stomach are rapidly emptied into the small intestine, causing dumping syndrome.
    - Early manifestations typically occur 15 to 30 min after eating. Late manifestations occur 1 to 3 hr after eating.
  - Early manifestations include a sensation of fullness, faintness, diaphoresis, tachycardia, palpitations, hypotension, nausea, abdominal distention, cramping pain, diarrhea, weakness, and syncope.
  - Manifestations resolve after intestine is emptied. However, there is a rapid rise in blood glucose and increase in insulin levels immediately after the intestine empties. This leads to hypoglycemia.
  - The client experiences vasomotor symptoms, such as dizziness, sweating, palpitations, shakiness, and confusion.
  - Nursing Interventions
    - Recommend small, frequent meals.
    - Recommend consumption of protein and fat at each meal.
    - Tell the client to avoid food that contains concentrated sugars and to restrict lactose intake.
    - Suggest that the client consume liquids 1 hr before or after eating instead of during meals (dry diet).
    - Instruct client to lie down for 20 to 30 min to after meals to delay gastric emptying. If reflux is a problem, assume a reclining position.
    - Monitor clients receiving enteral tube feedings and report clinical manifestations of dumping syndrome to the provider.
    - Monitor the client for vitamin and mineral deficits, such as iron and vitamin B_{12}.
- Gastroesophageal reflux disease (GERD)
  - GERD occurs as the result of the abnormal reflux of gastric secretions up the esophagus. This leads to indigestion and heartburn.
  - Long-term GERD can cause serious complications including adenocarcinoma of the esophagus and Barrett's esophagus.
  - Clinical manifestations include heartburn, retrosternal burning, painful swallowing, dyspepsia, regurgitation, coughing, hoarseness, and epigastric pain. Pain may be mistaken for a myocardial infarction.
  - Nursing Interventions
    - Instruct the client to avoid situations that lead to increased abdominal pressure, such as wearing tight-fitting clothing.
    - Advise the client to avoid eating 2 hr or less before lying down.
    - Advise the client to elevate the body on pillows instead of lying flat and to avoid large meals and bedtime snacks.
    - Encourage weight loss for overweight clients.

- Suggest that the client avoid trigger foods (citrus fruits and juices, spicy foods, carbonated beverages).
- Instruct the client to avoid items that reduce lower esophageal sphincter (LES) pressure, including fatty foods, caffeine, chocolate, alcohol, cigarette smoke and all nicotine products, and peppermint and spearmint flavors

- Acute and chronic gastritis
  - Gastritis is characterized by inflammation of the gastric mucosa. The gastric mucosa is congested with blood and fluid, becoming inflamed. There is a decrease in acid produced and an overabundance of mucus. Superficial ulcers occur, sometimes leading to hemorrhages.
  - Acute gastritis occurs with excessive use of NSAIDs, bile reflux, ingestion of a strong acid or alkali substance, as a complication of radiation therapy, or as a complication of trauma (burns; food poisoning; severe infection; liver, kidney, or respiratory failure; major surgery).
  - Chronic gastritis occurs in the presence of ulcers (benign or malignant), *Helicobacter pylori*, autoimmune disorders (pernicious anemia), poor diet (excessive caffeine, excessive alcohol intake), medications (alendronate [Fosamax], perindopril [Aceon]), and reflux of pancreatic secretions and bile into stomach.
  - Clinical manifestations include abdominal pain or discomfort (may be relieved by eating), headache, lassitude, nausea, anorexia, hiccupping (lasting a few hours to days), heartburn after eating, belching, sour taste in mouth, vomiting, bleeding, and hematemesis (vomiting of blood).
  - Nursing Interventions
    - Suggest that the client avoid eating frequent meals and snacks, as they promote increased gastric acid secretion.
    - Tell the client to avoid alcohol, cigarette smoking, aspirin and other nonsteroidal anti-inflammatory drugs (NSAIDs), coffee, black pepper, spicy foods, and caffeine.
    - Monitor the client for vitamin deficiency, especially of vitamin B_{12}.
  - Acute recovery typically occurs in 1 day, but may take 2 to 3 days. The client should eat bland diet when able to tolerate food. IV fluid replacement therapy may be required if the condition persists.
  - When the condition occurs due to ingestion of strong acids or alkalis, dilution and neutralization of the causal agent is needed. Avoid lavage and emetics due to potential perforation and esophageal damage.

  - Chronic management: modify diet, reduce and manage stress, avoid alcohol and NSAIDS. If condition is persistent, the provider will prescribe an H_2-receptor antagonist such as ranitidine (Zantac).

- Peptic ulcer disease (PUD)
  - PUD is characterized by an erosion of the mucosal layer of the stomach or duodenum.
  - This may be caused by a bacterial infection with *H. pylori* or the chronic use of NSAIDs (aspirin, ibuprofen).
  - Some clients who have PUD are asymptomatic. Others report dull, gnawing pain, burning sensation in the back or low midepigastric area, heartburn, constipation or diarrhea, sour taste in mouth, burping, nausea, vomiting, bloating, urea present in breath, and tarry stools. Eating may temporarily relieve pain. Anemia can occur due to blood loss.

- For PUD caused by *H. pylori*, the provider prescribes triple therapy (a combination of antibiotics and acid reducing medications) to be taken for 14 days.
- Nursing Interventions
  - Advise the client to avoid eating frequent meals and snacks as they promote increased gastric acid secretion.
  - Suggest that the client avoid coffee, alcohol, caffeine, aspirin and other NSAIDs, cigarette smoking, black pepper, and spicy foods.
- Lactose intolerance
  - Lactose intolerance results from an inadequate supply of lactase in the intestine, the enzyme that digests lactose.
  - The enzyme that converts lactose into glucose, and galactose is absent or insufficient. Clinical manifestations include distention, cramps, flatus, and osmotic diarrhea.
  - Nursing Interventions
    - Encourage clients to avoid or limit their intake of foods high in lactose (milk, cheese, ice cream, cream soups, sour cream, puddings, chocolate, coffee creamer).
    - Suggest that the client ask the provider about the use of a lactase enzyme.
    - Monitor the client for vitamin D deficiency and calcium.
- Ileostomies and colostomies
  - An ostomy is a surgically created opening on the surface of the abdomen from either the end of the small intestine (ileostomy) or from the colon (colostomy).
  - Fluid and electrolyte maintenance is the primary concern for clients who have ileostomies and colostomies.
  - The colon absorbs large amounts of fluid, sodium, and potassium.
  - Nutrition therapy begins with liquids only and is slowly advanced based upon client tolerance.
  - Nursing Interventions
    - Advise the client to consume a diet that is high in fluids and soluble fiber.
    - Encourage the client to avoid foods that cause gas (beans, eggs, carbonated beverages), stomal blockage (nuts, raw carrots, popcorn), and foods that produce odor (eggs, fish, garlic).
    - Encourage the client to increase his intake of calories and protein to promote healing of the stoma site.

    - Provide emotional support to clients due to their altered body image.
- Diverticulosis and diverticulitis
  - Diverticula are pouches protruding through the muscle of the intestinal wall, usually from increased intraluminal pressure. They occur anywhere in the colon, but usually in the sigmoid colon. Unless infection occurs, diverticula cause no problems.
  - Diverticulosis is a condition characterized by the presence of diverticula.
  - Diverticulitis is inflammation that occurs when fecal matter becomes trapped in the diverticula.
  - Clinical manifestations of diverticulitis include abdominal pain, nausea, vomiting, constipation or diarrhea, and fever, accompanied by chills and tachycardia.

- The client is administered antibiotics, anticholinergics, and analgesics. Clients who have severe manifestations are admitted to the hospital and dehydration is treated with IV therapy. Opioid analgesics are administered for pain. Complications (peritonitis, bowel obstruction, abscess) may warrant surgical intervention.

- A high-fiber diet may prevent diverticulosis and diverticulitis by producing stools that are easily passed, thus decreasing pressure within the colon.

- During acute diverticulitis, a clear liquid diet is prescribed until inflammation decreases, then a high-fiber, low-fat diet is indicated.

- Instruct the client to avoid foods with seeds or husks (corn, popcorn, berries, tomatoes).

- Clients require instruction regarding diet adjustment based on the need for an acute intervention or preventive approach.

- Inflammatory bowel disease

  - Crohn's disease (regional enteritis) and ulcerative colitis are chronic, inflammatory bowel diseases characterized by periods of exacerbation and remission.

  - Clinical manifestations include nausea, vomiting, abdominal cramps, fever, fatigue, anorexia, weight loss, steatorrhea, and low-grade fever.

  - Nutrition therapy is focused on providing nutrients in forms that the client can tolerate.

  - Generally, diets are low in fiber to minimize bowel stimulation.

  - A low-residue, high-protein, high-calorie diet with vitamin and mineral supplementation is prescribed. Fluid and electrolyte imbalances are corrected with IV fluids or oral replacement fluids.

  - Teach clients to avoid intake of substances that cause or exacerbate diarrhea, and to avoid nicotine.

  - Total parenteral nutrition (TPN) is indicated for clients who are severely ill during the acute phase of the illness.

  - Additional therapy

    - Sedatives

    - Antidiarrheal and antiperistaltic agents

    - Aminosalicylate medications and corticosteroids to reduce inflammation

    - Immunomodulators to alter the immune response and prevent relapse

    - Surgery when other treatments are not effective

- Cholecystitis

  - Cholecystitis is characterized by inflammation of the gallbladder.

  - The gallbladder stores and releases bile that aids in the digestion of fats.

  - Clinical manifestations include pain, tenderness, and rigidity in upper right abdomen. Pain can radiate to the right shoulder or midsternal area. Nausea, vomiting, and anorexia also can occur. If the gallbladder becomes filled with pus or becomes gangrenous, perforation can result.

  - In clients who have large stones or inability to control the condition with diet modifications, surgery is required.

  - Pancreatitis and liver involvement can result from uncontrolled cholecystitis.

  - Fat intake should be limited to reduce stimulation of the gallbladder.

- ○ Other foods that may cause problems include coffee, broccoli, cauliflower, Brussels sprouts, cabbage, onions, legumes, and highly seasoned foods.

- ○ The diet is individualized to the client's needs and tolerance.

- ○ Diet modifications are not necessary for healthy people with asymptomatic gallstones.

- Pancreatitis

  - ○ Pancreatitis is an inflammation of the pancreas.

  - ○ The pancreas is responsible for secreting enzymes needed to digest fats, carbohydrates, and proteins.

  - ○ Nutritional therapy for acute pancreatitis involves reducing pancreatic stimulation. The client is prescribed nothing by mouth (NPO), and a nasogastric tube is inserted to suction gastric contents.

  - ○ TPN may be used until oral intake is resumed.

  - ○ Nutritional therapy for chronic pancreatitis usually includes a low-fat, high-protein, and high-carbohydrate diet. It may include providing supplements of vitamin C and B-complex vitamins.

- Liver disease

  - ○ The liver is involved in the metabolism of almost all nutrients.

  - ○ Disorders affecting the liver include cirrhosis, hepatitis, and cancer.

  - ○ Malnutrition is common with liver disease.

  - ○ Protein needs are increased to promote a positive nitrogen balance and to prevent a breakdown of the body's protein stores.

  - ○ Carbohydrates are generally not restricted, as they are an important source of calories.

  - ○ Caloric requirements may need to be increased based upon an evaluation of the client's stage of disease, weight, and general health status.

  - ○ Multivitamins (especially vitamins B, C, and K) and mineral supplements may be necessary.

  - ○ Alcohol, nicotine, and caffeine should be eliminated.

- Celiac disease

  - ○ Celiac disease is also known as gluten-sensitive enteropathy (GSE), celiac sprue, and gluten intolerance.

  - ○ It is a chronic, inherited, genetic disorder with autoimmune characteristics. Clients who have celiac disease are unable to digest the protein gluten. They lack the digestive enzyme DPP-IV, which is required to break down the gluten into molecules small enough to be used by the body. In celiac disease, gluten is broken down into peptide strands instead molecules. The body is not able to metabolize the peptides. If untreated, the client will suffer destruction of the villa and the walls of the small intestine. Celiac disease may go undiagnosed in both children and adults.

  - ○ Clinical manifestations vary widely. Children who have celiac disease have diarrhea, steatorrhea, anemia, abdominal distention, impaired growth, lack of appetite, and fatigue. Typical manifestations in adults include diarrhea, abdominal pain, bloating, anemia, steatorrhea, and osteomalacia.

○ Treatment for celiac disease is limited to avoiding gluten. However, eliminating gluten, which is found in wheat, rye and barley, is difficult because it is found in many prepared foods. Clients must read food labels carefully in order to adhere to a gluten-free diet. Some gluten-free products are unappealing to clients, and many are more expensive that other products. Prognosis is good for clients who adhere to a gluten-free diet.

○ Nursing Interventions

  ▪ Encourage clients to eat foods that are gluten-free: milk, cheese, rice, corn, eggs, potatoes, fruits, vegetables, fresh poultry, meats and fish, dried beans.

  ▪ Remind clients to read labels on processed products. Gravy mixes, sauces, cold cuts, soups, and many other products have gluten as an ingredient. Advise clients to read labels on nonfood products, which also may have gluten as an ingredient.

APPLICATION EXERCISES

1. A nurse is providing dietary instructions to a client who is recovering from acute gastroenteritis and has been advised to limit his intake to low-fat foods. The nurse should suggest that the client eat which of the following foods? (Select all that apply.)

_____ A. Saltine crackers

_____ B. Oatmeal

_____ C. Ice cream

_____ D. Canned peaches

_____ E. Pretzels

2. A nurse is providing instructions to a client who reports constipation and has a prescription for a high-fiber, low-fat diet. Which of the following food choices by the client indicates he understands the teaching?

A. Peanut butter

B. Peeled apples

C. Hardboiled egg

D. Brown rice

3. A nurse is assessing a client who is postoperative from a gastric bypass and who just finished a meal. Which of the following clinical findings are early indications of dumping syndrome? (Select all that apply.)

_____ A. Bradycardia

_____ B. Dizziness

_____ C. Dry skin

_____ D. Hypotension

_____ E. Diarrhea

4. A nurse is obtaining an admission history from a client who is being evaluated for peptic ulcer disease (PUD). Which of the following findings are indicative of this condition? (Select all that apply.)

_____ A. Steatorrhea

_____ B. Anemia

_____ C. Tarry stools

_____ D. Epigastric pain

_____ E. Swollen lymph nodes

5. A nurse is providing instructions to a client who has a new diagnosis of celiac disease. Which of the following food choices by the client indicates a need for further teaching?

    A. Potatoes

    B. Graham crackers

    C. Wild rice

    D. Canned pears

6. A nurse is providing instructions to the parent of a child who has lactose intolerance. What should the nurse include in the teaching? Use the ATI Active Learning Template: Systems Disorder to complete this item to include the following:

    A. Client Education:

      • Describe the underlying cause of lactose intolerance.

      • Identify two clinical manifestations of lactose intolerance.

      • Identify three foods the child should limit or eliminate from his diet.

APPLICATION EXERCISES KEY

1. A. **CORRECT:** Saltine crackers are a source of easily digested carbohydrate that is low in fat.

    B. **CORRECT:** Oatmeal is a source of easily digested carbohydrate that is low in fat.

    C. INCORRECT: One third cup of ice cream contains 7 grams of fat.

    D. **CORRECT:** Canned peaches are a source of easily digested carbohydrate that is low in fat.

    E. **CORRECT:** Pretzels are a source of easily digested carbohydrate that is low in fat.

    Ⓝ NCLEX® Connection: Basic Care and Comfort, Nutrition and Oral Hydration

2. A. INCORRECT: Peanut butter is high in fat. This choice indicates that the client does not understand the teaching.

    B. INCORRECT: Unpeeled fruit is a better source of fiber. This choice indicates that the client does not understand the teaching.

    C. INCORRECT: Egg yolk is high in fat. This choice indicates that the client does not understand the teaching.

    D. **CORRECT:** Brown rice is a good source of fiber and is low in fat. This choice indicates that the client understands the teaching.

    Ⓝ NCLEX® Connection: Basic Care and Comfort, Elimination

3. A. INCORRECT: When a portion of the stomach is no longer available to serve as a reservoir, a large amount of food is rapidly dumped into the small intestine, and fluid shifts from general circulation into the intestine. Tachycardia occurs due to a decrease in circulating volume.

    B. **CORRECT:** When a portion of the stomach is no longer available to serve as a reservoir, a large amount of food is rapidly dumped into the small intestine, and fluid shifts from general circulation into the intestine. Dizziness occurs due to a decrease in circulating volume.

    C. INCORRECT: Sweating, not dry skin, is a clinical manifestation of dumping syndrome.

    D. **CORRECT:** When a portion of the stomach is no longer available to serve as a reservoir, a large amount of food is rapidly dumped into the small intestine, and fluid shifts from general circulation into the intestine. Hypotension occurs due to a decrease in circulating volume.

    E. **CORRECT:** When a portion of the stomach is no longer available to serve as a reservoir, a large amount of food is rapidly dumped into the small intestine, which causes increased peristalsis, and diarrhea occurs.

    Ⓝ NCLEX® Connection: Basic Care and Comfort, Elimination

4. A. INCORRECT: Steatorrhea is a clinical finding in the presence celiac disease.

    B. **CORRECT:** Iron deficiency anemia due to blood loss is a clinical finding of PUD.

    C. **CORRECT:** Tarry stools due to intestinal bleeding is a clinical finding of PUD.

    D. **CORRECT:** Epigastric pain described as a gnawing or burning sensation is a clinical manifestation of PUD.

    E. INCORRECT: Swollen lymph nodes are a clinical manifestation of many conditions and infections, but not of PUD.

    ⓝ NCLEX® Connection: Basic Care and Comfort, Elimination

5. A. INCORRECT: Potatoes are gluten-free and a good choice for a client who has celiac disease.

    B. **CORRECT:** Graham crackers are made from wheat flour. A client who has celiac disease should avoid products that are made from wheat flour.

    C. INCORRECT: Wild rice is gluten-free and a good choice for a client who has celiac disease.

    D. INCORRECT: Fruits and vegetable without a sauce are gluten-free and a good choice for a client who has celiac disease.

    ⓝ NCLEX® Connection: Basic Care and Comfort, Nutrition and Oral Hydration

6. *Using the ATI Active Learning Template: Systems Disorder*

    A. Client Education
        • Lactose intolerance is due to an inadequate level of lactase. The enzyme that converts lactose into glucose and galactose is absent or insufficient.
        • Clinical Manifestations
            ○ Abdominal distension
            ○ Cramps
            ○ Flatus
            ○ Diarrhea
        • Foods to limit or avoid: milk, cheese, ice cream, cream soups, puddings, chocolate.

    ⓝ NCLEX® Connection: Physiological Adaptations, Illness Management

chapter 14

Overview

- Nurses must gain an awareness of nutritional needs for clients who have renal disorders. It is important to explore dietary needs with the client and recommend modifications in relationship to the disease process. Understanding the role of primary and secondary prevention is essential to successful treatment.

- Specific nutritional considerations covered in this chapter are:
  - Pre-stage chronic kidney disease
  - End-stage kidney disease or chronic kidney disease
  - Acute kidney failure
  - Nephrotic syndrome
  - Nephrolithiasis (kidney stones)

- The kidneys have two basic functions: maintaining normal blood volume and excreting waste products.
  - Kidney damage and/or loss of kidney function has profound effects on the nutritional state.
  - Urea is a waste by-product of protein metabolism, and urea levels rise with renal disease. Monitoring protein intake is paramount for clients who have renal disease.

- Short-term kidney disease requires nutritional support for healing rather than dietary restrictions. Dietary recommendations are dependent upon the stage of kidney disease.

Assessment/Data Collection

- Pre-stage chronic kidney disease (CKD) is distinguished by an increase in serum creatinine. Manifestations include fatigue, back pain, and appetite changes.

- End-stage kidney disease (ESKD) or CKD manifestations include fatigue, decreased alertness, anemia, decreased urination, headache, and weight loss.

- Acute kidney injury (AKI) manifestations include a decrease in urination, decreased sensation in the extremities, swelling of the lower extremities, and flank pain. It is characterized by rising blood levels of urea and other nitrogenous wastes.

- Nephrotic syndrome's most pronounced manifestations are edema and high proteinuria. Other manifestations include hypoalbuminemia, hyperlipidemia, and blood hypercoagulation.

- Kidney stone is characterized by sudden, intense pain that is typically located in the flank and is unrelieved by position changes as the stone moves out of the kidney pelvis and down the ureter. Diaphoresis, nausea, and vomiting are common, and there can be blood in the urine. Approximately 80% of stones contain calcium.

Nutritional Guidelines and Nursing Interventions

- General Renal Considerations
  - ○ Monitor kidney parameters for clients who have renal disorders.
    - ▪ Nurses should monitor weight daily or as prescribed. Weight is an indicator of fluid status, which is a primary concern.
    - ▪ Monitor fluid intake and encourage compliance with fluid restrictions.
    - ▪ Nurses should monitor urine output. Placement of an indwelling urinary catheter may be necessary for accurate measurement.
    - ▪ Monitor for manifestations of constipation. Fluid restrictions predispose clients to constipation.
  - ○ Explain why dietary changes are necessary. Ultimately, alterations in the intake of protein, calories, sodium, potassium, phosphorus, and other vitamins will be needed.
  - ○ Provide support for the client and family.
- Pre-stage CKD
  - ○ Pre-stage CKD, or diminished kidney reserve/kidney insufficiency, is a predialysis condition characterized by an increase in serum creatinine.
  - ○ Therapeutic Nutrition
    - ▪ Goals of nutritional therapy to slow the progression of pre-stage CKD are to:
      - □ Control blood glucose and hypertension, which are risk factors.
      - □ Help preserve remaining kidney function by limiting the intake of protein and phosphorus.
    - ▪ Restricting phosphorus intake slows the progression of kidney disease.
      - □ High levels of phosphorus contribute to calcium and phosphorus deposits in the kidneys.
    - ▪ Protein restriction is essential for clients who have pre-stage CKD.
      - □ Slows the progression of kidney disease.
      - □ Too little protein results in the breakdown of body protein. Protein intake must be carefully determined.
    - ▪ Dietary recommendations for pre-stage CKD
      - □ Restrict sodium intake to maintain blood pressure.
      - □ The recommended daily protein intake is 0.6 to 1.0 g/kg of ideal body weight. Protein restrictions are decreased as the disease progresses to end-stage CKD, and to decrease the workload on the kidneys.
        - ▸ High biologic value proteins are recommended for clients who have kidney failure to prevent catabolism of muscle tissue. These proteins include eggs, meats, poultry, game, fish, soy, and dairy products.
      - □ Limit meat intake to 5 to 6 oz/day for most men and 4 oz/day for most women.
      - □ Limit dairy products to ½ cup per day.

- □ Limit high-phosphorus foods (peanut butter, dried peas and beans, bran, cola, chocolate, beer, some whole grains) to one serving or less per day.
- □ Caution clients to use vitamin and mineral supplements only when recommended by a health care provider. Avoid sports drinks, energy drinks, or meal supplement systems, which can be high-protein. Avoid herbal supplements that may affect bleeding time and blood pressure.

- End-stage kidney disease (ESKD)
  - ESKD or CKD occurs when the glomerular filtration rate (GFR) is less than 29 mL/min, the serum creatinine level steadily rises, or dialysis or transplantation is necessary.
  - Therapeutic Nutrition
    - The goal of nutritional therapy is to maintain appropriate fluid status, blood pressure, and blood chemistries.
      - □ A high-protein, low-phosphorus, low-potassium, low-sodium (2 to 4 g/day), fluid-restricted diet is recommended.
      - □ Once dialysis begins, protein intake will be increased because some protein is lost during dialysis. The amount of protein increase will depend on whether hemodialysis or peritoneal dialysis is being performed.
      - □ Vitamin D and calcium are nutrients of concern.
    - Potassium intake is dependent upon the client's laboratory findings, which should be closely monitored.
    - Sodium and fluid allowances are determined by blood pressure, weight, serum electrolyte findings, and urine output.
    - Achieving a well-balanced diet based on the above guidelines is difficult. The National Renal Diet provides clients with a list of appropriate food choices.
    - Protein needs increase once dialysis has begun as protein and amino acids are lost in the dialysate.
      - □ Fifty percent of protein intake should come from biologic sources (eggs, milk, meat, fish, poultry, soy).
      - □ Adequate calories (35 kcal/kg of body weight) should be consumed to maintain body protein stores.
    - Phosphorus must be restricted.
      - □ A high protein requirement leads to an increase in phosphorus intake.
      - □ Foods high in phosphorus are milk products, beef liver, chocolate, nuts, and legumes.
      - □ Phosphate binders (e.g., calcium carbonate, calcium acetate) must be taken with all meals and snacks.
    - Vitamin D deficiency occurs as the kidneys are unable to convert vitamin D to its active form.
      - □ This alters the metabolism of calcium, phosphorus, and magnesium, leading to hyperphosphatemia, hypocalcemia, and hypermagnesemia.
      - □ Calcium supplements will likely be required because foods high in phosphorus (which are restricted) are also high in calcium.

- Acute kidney injury (AKI)
  - AKI is an abrupt, rapid decline in kidney function caused by trauma, sepsis, poor perfusion, or medications, and usually is reversible. AKI can cause hyponatremia, hyperkalemia, hypocalcemia, and hyperphosphatemia. Infection is a complication of AKI and is the leading cause of death in these clients.
  - Therapeutic Nutrition
    - Diet therapy for AKI is dependent upon the phase of AKI and its underlying cause. Protein, calories, fluids, potassium, and sodium need to be individualized according to the three phases of AKI (oliguric phase, diuretic phase, and recovery phase), and adjusted as improvement develops if the client is receiving dialysis.
    - Recommendation is to consume 30 to 50 kcal/kg of body weight to maintain energy and demands of stress.
    - Simple carbohydrates, fats, oils, and low-protein starches provide nonprotein calories.
    - Protein intake may increase if the client is receiving dialysis, from 0.6 to 2 g/kg compared to 0.6 g/kg (40 g/day) for nondialysis clients.
    - Potassium and sodium are dependent on urine output, serum values, and if the client is receiving dialysis.
      - Potassium is restricted to 60 to 70 mEq/day when on dialysis.
      - Sodium is restricted to 1 to 3 g/day if not receiving dialysis, and 1 to 4 g/day if receiving dialysis, which also depends on the phase.
      - Calcium requirements are of less than 2,000 mg daily if on hemodialysis or peritoneal dialysis.
    - Fluids are restricted to the client's daily urine output plus 500 mL during the oliguric phase. Fluid needs are increased during the diuretic phase.
- Nephrotic syndrome
  - Nephrotic syndrome results in the increased excretion of serum proteins into the urine, resulting in hypoalbuminemia, edema, hyperlipidemia, and blood hypercoagulation. Prolonged protein loss leads to protein malnutrition, anemia, and vitamin D deficiency.
  - Diabetes mellitus, kidney damage due to medications or chemicals, autoimmune disorders, and infections can cause nephrotic syndrome.
  - Therapeutic Nutrition
    - Nutritional therapy goals include minimizing edema, replacing lost nutrients, minimizing renal damage, controlling hypertension, and preventing protein malnutrition that can lead to muscle catabolism.
    - Dietary recommendations indicate sufficient protein and low sodium intake.
      - Adequate amount of protein intake is 0.7 to 1.0 g/kg/day.
      - Soy-based proteins may decrease protein losses and lower serum lipid levels.
      - Low-sodium diet of 1,000 to 2,000 mg can help control edema and hypertension.
      - Carbohydrates should provide the majority of the client's daily calories.
      - Foods high in trans fats and cholesterol are limited, and total fat should be less than 30% of the daily diet.
      - Provide a multiple vitamin supplement to replace loss of vitamins with protein excretion.

- Nephrolithiasis (kidney stones)
  - Most common type of kidney stone is made of calcium oxalate.
  - Contributing factors include inadequate fluid intake, elevated urine pH, and excess excretion through the kidneys of oxalate, calcium, and uric acid.
  - Kidney stone formation is more influenced by the amount of oxalate in the client's system than calcium. A client who has an ileostomy has a higher incidence of kidney stones.
  - Preventative Nutrition
    - Excessive intake of protein, sodium, calcium, and oxalates (rhubarb, spinach, beets) may increase the risk of stone formation.
  - Therapeutic Nutrition
    - Increasing fluid consumption is the primary intervention for the treatment and prevention of kidney stones. Daily fluid intake should be at least 1,500 mL to 3,000 mL. At least 8 to 12 oz (240 to 360 mL) of fluid, preferably water, should be consumed before bedtime because urine becomes more concentrated at night.
    - Recommendation for calcium oxalate stone formation is to limit animal protein, excess sodium, alcohol, and caffeine use. Low potassium also may be a contributing factor in calcium stone formation.
    - Foods high in oxalates include spinach, rhubarb, beets, nuts, chocolate, tea, wheat bran, and strawberries and should be limited in the diet. Avoid megadoses of vitamin C, which increases the amount of oxalate excreted.
    - Recommendation for prevention of uric acid stones is to limit foods high in purines, which include lean meats, organ meats, whole grains, and legumes.

APPLICATION EXERCISES

1. A nurse is planning care for a client who has chronic kidney disease. Which of the following should the nurse include in the plan of care? (Select all that apply.)

_____ A. Monitor daily weights.

_____ B. Encourage compliance with fluid restrictions.

_____ C. Evaluate intake and output.

_____ D. Instruct on restricting calories from carbohydrates.

_____ E. Monitor for constipation.

2. A nurse is teaching a client who has pre-stage chronic kidney disease about dietary management. Which of the following information should the nurse include in the instructions?

A. Restrict protein intake.

B. Maintain a high-phosphorus diet.

C. Increase intake of foods high in potassium.

D. Limit dairy products to 1 cup per day.

3. A nurse is teaching a client about protein needs when on dialysis. Which of the following should the nurse include in the teaching? (Select all that apply.)

_____ A. Consume 35 kcal/kg of body weight.

_____ B. Eating high-protein foods leads to increased phosphorus intake.

_____ C. Biologic sources of protein are eggs, milk, and soy.

_____ D. Amino acids are lost in the dialysate.

_____ E. Protein needs decrease once dialysis is started.

4. A nurse is teaching about diet restrictions to a client who has acute kidney injury and is on hemodialysis. Which of the following should the nurse include in the teaching?

A. Limit calcium intake to 2,500 mg daily.

B. Decrease total fat intake to 45% of daily calories.

C. Decrease potassium intake to 65 mEq/day.

D. Limit sodium intake to 4.5 g/day.

5. A nurse is completing discharge teaching about diet and fluid restrictions to a client who has a calcium-oxalate based kidney stone. Which of the following should the nurse include in the teaching?

    A. Reduce intake of strawberries.

    B. Decease broccoli intake.

    C. Increase intake of juices rich in vitamin C.

    D. Limit consumption of whole-grain foods.

6. A nurse is reviewing teaching for a client who has nephrotic syndrome. What information should the nurse include? Use the ATI Active Learning Template: System Disorder to complete this item to include the following:

    A. Description of Disorder/Disease Process

    B. Potential Complication: List three.

    C. Management of Client Care: Include five teaching points.

APPLICATION EXERCISES KEY

1. A. **CORRECT:** Monitoring daily weight assists in determining fluid retention.

    B. **CORRECT:** Implementing fluid restrictions helps to slow fluid retention.

    C. **CORRECT:** Evaluating I&O helps to determine if there is an increase in fluid retention.

    D. INCORRECT: Protein is restricted for a client who has chronic kidney disease.

    E. **CORRECT:** Constipation often occurs as a result of fluid restrictions.

    Ⓝ NCLEX® Connection: Basic Care and Comfort, Nutrition and Oral Hydration

2. A. **CORRECT:** Restricting protein intake decreases the workload on the kidney.

    B. INCORRECT: A diet high in phosphorus is not recommended because it can contribute to calcium and phosphorus deposits on the kidney.

    C. INCORRECT: Eating foods low in potassium is recommended because hyperkalemia occurs with kidney disease.

    D. INCORRECT: Dairy products are a protein and sodium source, and are limited to 0.5 cup/day.

    Ⓝ NCLEX® Connection: Basic Care and Comfort, Nutrition and Oral Hydration

3. A. **CORRECT:** To maintain protein stores, the client should consume 35 kcal/kg of body weight.

    B. **CORRECT:** Protein consumption increases phosphorus intake. Phosphate binders are recommended with meals.

    C. **CORRECT:** Protein intake should include biologic sources of protein to include eggs, milk, meat, fish, poultry, and soy.

    D. **CORRECT:** Amino acids are protein and are lost in the dialysate.

    E. INCORRECT: Protein needs increase with dialysis.

    Ⓝ NCLEX® Connection: Basic Care and Comfort, Nutrition and Oral Hydration

4. A. INCORRECT: The client receiving hemodialysis should limit calcium intake to less than 2,000 mg/day.

    B. INCORRECT: The client's total fat intake should be limited to 30% of daily calories.

    C. **CORRECT:** The client's potassium intake should be restricted to 60 to 70 mEq/day.

    D. INCORRECT: The client's sodium intake should be restricted to 1 to 4 g/day when receiving dialysis.

    Ⓝ NCLEX® Connection: Basic Care and Comfort, Nutrition and Oral Hydration

5. A. **CORRECT:** Foods high in oxalate include strawberries, which can cause calcium stone formation and should be limited in the diet.

    B. INCORRECT: Broccoli is high in calcium but does not cause calcium stone formation and is not restricted in the diet.

    C. INCORRECT: Juices rich in vitamin C and vitamin C supplements can cause calcium stone formation and should be limited in the diet.

    D. INCORRECT: Whole-grain foods are restricted in a low-purine diet and cause uric acid stone formation.

    Ⓝ NCLEX® Connection: Health Promotion and Maintenance, Health Promotion/Disease Prevention

6. *Using the ATI Active Learning Template: System Disorder*

    A. Description of Disorder/Disease Process
    - Nephrotic syndrome is a renal disorder in which there is increased excretion of serum proteins into the urine.

    B. Potential Complications
    - Hypoalbuminemia
    - Edema
    - Hyperlipidemia
    - Malnutrition

    C. Management of Client Care
    - Increase protein intake to prevent catabolism of muscle tissue.
    - Limit sodium intake to control edema and hypertension.
    - Consume foods low in trans fats and cholesterol.
    - Consume foods high in carbohydrates to increase calorie intake.
    - Take a vitamin supplement to replace vitamin loss that occurs with protein excretion.

    Ⓝ NCLEX® Connection: Physiological Adaptations, Illness Management

NUTRITION FOR NURSING

chapter 15

Overview

- Nurses must gain an awareness of nutritional needs for clients who have diabetes mellitus. It is important to explore dietary needs with the client and recommend modifications in relationship to the disease process. Understanding the role of primary and secondary prevention is essential to successful management.
- Diabetes mellitus inhibits the body's production and/or use of insulin. This results in above-normal glucose levels and health complications including heart disease, blindness, kidney failure, and deterioration and decreased function of nerves.
  - ○ Glucose is the body's primary source of energy, and insulin is needed to assist the body in the breakdown of glucose to a form that can be used by the body for energy.
  - ○ The goal of management is to assist the client in making the appropriate lifestyle changes and nutritional choices necessary to control blood glucose levels.
  - ○ Achieving proper nutrition and meeting specific dietary needs is essential in controlling the effects of diabetes mellitus.
  - ○ Blood glucose levels are used to diagnose diabetes.
- Types of Diabetes Mellitus
  - ○ Type 1 Diabetes Mellitus
    - Autoimmune disease triggered by genetic links or a viral infection.
    - Damage to or destruction of beta cells of the pancreas results in an absence of insulin production.
    - Usually occurs in individuals under the age of 30 with a normal or below-normal weight.
  - ○ Type 2 Diabetes Mellitus
    - Results from genetic and environmental factors.
    - Characterized by altered patterns of insulin secretion and decreased cellular uptake of glucose (insulin resistance).
    - Usually occurs in individuals over the age of 40.
    - Obesity and sedentary lifestyle are risk factors.
  - ○ Gestational Diabetes Mellitus (GDM)
    - Glucose intolerance that is recognized during pregnancy.
    - Usually occurs during the second and third trimesters.
    - Occurs only during pregnancy and typically resolves after delivery.
    - Characterized by increased insulin resistance caused by secretion of placental hormones, and increased insulin antagonists.
    - Many women with GDM develop type 2 diabetes mellitus later in life.
    - Blood glucose control is important in preventing damage to the fetus of women who are pregnant and who have GDM or pre-existing diabetes mellitus.

Assessment/Data Collection

- Hypoglycemia is an abnormally low blood glucose level.

  - It results from taking too much insulin, inadequate food intake, delayed or skipped meals, extra physical activity, or consumption of alcohol without food.

  - Blood glucose of 70 mg/dL or less requires immediate action.

  - Manifestations include mild shakiness, mental confusion, sweating, palpitations, headache, lack of coordination, blurred vision, seizures, and coma.

- Hyperglycemia is an abnormally high blood glucose level.

  - It results from an imbalance among food, medication, and activity.

  - Infection, other illness, and stress can cause a rise in blood glucose.

  - Manifestations include blood glucose greater than 250 mg/dL, ketones in urine, polydipsia (excessive thirst), polyuria (excessive urination), polyphagia (excess hunger and eating), hyperventilation (Kussmaul respirations), dehydration, fruity odor to breath, headache, inability to concentrate, decreased levels of consciousness, and seizures leading to coma.

Nutritional Guidelines and Nursing Interventions

- Hypoglycemia

  - Clients with hypoglycemia should be instructed to take 15 to 20 g of a readily absorbable carbohydrate, such as:

    - Two or three glucose tablets (5 g each).

    - Eight Lifesavers™/hard candies.

    - ½ cup (4 oz) juice or regular soda.

    - 1 tbsp of honey or brown sugar.

  - Retest the blood glucose in 15 min. If it is less than 70 mg/dL, repeat the above steps. Once levels normalize, have the client take an additional carbohydrate and protein snack or small meal, depending on the severity of the hypoglycemic episode and whether the next meal is more than 1 hr away.

- Hyperglycemia

  - Clients with hyperglycemia should:

    - Immediately consult a provider, or go to the emergency department.

    - Take medication if forgotten.

    - Consider modifications to insulin or oral diabetic medications.

  - Long-term implications of untreated or inadequately treated hyperglycemia include blindness, kidney failure, dyslipidemia, hypertension, neuropathy, microvascular disease, and limb amputation.

  - Somogyi's phenomenon is morning hyperglycemia in response to overnight hypoglycemia. Providing a bedtime snack and appropriate insulin dose prevents this phenomenon.

  - Dawn phenomenon is an elevation of blood glucose around 0500 to 0600. It results from an overnight release of growth hormone, and is treated by increasing the amount of insulin provided during the overnight hours.

- General Nutritional Guidelines
  - Coronary heart disease (CHD) is the leading cause of death among clients who have diabetes. Therefore, clients who have diabetes are encouraged to follow a diet that is high in fiber and low in saturated fat, trans fat, and cholesterol.
  - Dietary intake should be individualized according to the client's food intake, need for weight management, and lipid and glucose patterns. General guidelines include:
    - Carbohydrates
      - ▫ Encourage the client to consume carbohydrates found in grains, fruits, legumes, and milk. Limit simple carbohydrates, which include refined grains and sugars.
        - ▸ Carbohydrates should include a minimum of 130 g/day for healthy brain function.
        - ▸ Carbohydrates should be 45% to 60% of total daily caloric intake.
    - Fats
      - ▫ Saturated fat should account for less than 7% of total calories.
      - ▫ Trans fatty acid recommendation is less than 1% of total daily caloric intake. Limit fried foods and bakery products, which contain high quantities of trans fatty acid from preparation with hydrogenated oils.
      - ▫ Cholesterol is restricted to 200 to 300 mg/day.
      - ▫ Polyunsaturated fatty acids are found in fish. Two or more servings per week are recommended.
    - Fiber
      - ▫ Promote fiber intake (beans, vegetables, oats, whole grains) to improve carbohydrate metabolism and lower cholesterol.
      - ▫ Recommendation for fiber intake includes at least 14 g per 1,000 calories.
    - Protein
      - ▫ Protein from meats, eggs, fish, nuts, beans, and soy products should comprise 15% to 20% of total caloric intake. Protein intake may need to be reduced in clients who have diabetes and kidney failure.
  - Encourage clients with diabetes mellitus to eliminate all tobacco use due to the increased risk of cardiovascular disease.
  - Recommended maximum daily alcohol consumption for a client who has well-controlled diabetes is one alcoholic beverage for women or two for men.
    - To avoid hypoglycemia, the client should consume alcohol with a meal or immediately after a meal.
    - Alcohol is not recommended for a client who has hyperlipidemia.
    - Alcoholic beverages should replace two fat exchanges in the diabetic diet.
  - Vitamin and mineral requirements are unchanged for clients who have diabetes. Supplements are recommended for identified deficiencies. Deficiencies in magnesium and potassium can aggravate glucose intolerance.
  - Artificial sweeteners are acceptable. Saccharin crosses the placenta and should be avoided during pregnancy.
    - Sucrose (table sugar) can be included in a diabetic diet as long as adequate insulin or other agents are provided to cover the sugar intake.

- ○ Cultural and personal preferences should be considered in planning food intake.
- ○ According to the American Diabetes Association and the American Dietetic Association, daily nutritional requirements are based on the needs of each client.
  - ▪ The dietitian works with the client to develop meal planning that meets the client's needs based on healthy food choices.
  - ▪ The goal of therapy is to maintain blood glucose levels as close to the expected reference range as possible.
  - ▪ The dietitian instructs the client on various dietary methods, including exchange list and carbohydrate counting.
- ○ Using the exchange list as a guide for meal planning allows for the incorporation of three basic food groups: protein, carbohydrates, and fats.
  - ▪ This dietary regimen assists the client in maintaining a blood glucose level within a target range.
  - ▪ Each client has a recommended amount of daily exchanges within each group based on the client's needs.
- ○ Carbohydrate counting focuses on counting total grams of carbohydrates in each food item.
  - ▪ Each client is prescribed a number of grams of carbohydrates for each meal and daily snacks.
  - ▪ The dietitian determines the needs of the individual and provides instructions for reading food labels and counting carbohydrate amounts in food selections.
  - ▪ Carbohydrates can be exchanged as long as the portion size remains accurate.
- • Other Nursing Interventions
  - ○ Encourage exercise. Blood glucose and medication dosages should be closely monitored.
  - ○ Encourage weight loss. It is more important for clients with type 2 diabetes mellitus as it can decrease insulin resistance, improve glucose and lipid levels, and lower blood pressure.
  - ○ Clients should be encouraged to perform self-monitoring of blood glucose. Strict control of glucose can reduce or postpone complications (retinopathy, nephropathy, neuropathy).
    - ▪ Teach proper calibration and use of the self-monitoring of blood glucose, record keeping, and reporting of levels to health care provider.
  - ○ Clients should be encouraged to receive regular evaluations from the provider.
  - ○ Client education and support should be provided for:
    - ▪ Self-monitoring of blood glucose.
    - ▪ Dietary and activity recommendations.
    - ▪ Manifestations and treatment of hypoglycemia and hyperglycemia, to include the importance of taking medications as prescribed.
    - ▪ Long-term complications of diabetes
    - ▪ Psychological implications.
    - ▪ Community organizations and support groups whose focus is diabetes.
  - ○ Children who have diabetes require parental support, guidance, and participation. Dietary intake must provide for proper growth and development.

APPLICATION EXERCISES

1. A nurse is providing information to a client who has a new diagnosis of type 1 diabetes mellitus. Which of the following information should the nurse include? (Select all that apply.)

_____ A. It is triggered by a viral infection.

_____ B. Alpha cells in the pancreas are damaged.

_____ C. It usually occurs before age 30.

_____ D. It is treated with antiglycemic medications.

_____ E. Blood glucose is controlled by diet and exercise.

2. A nurse is assessing a client who has hypoglycemia. Which of the following findings should the nurse expect?

A. Fruity breath odor

B. Diaphoresis

C. Vomiting

D. Polyuria

3. A nurse is caring for a client who has hypoglycemia. Which of the following is an appropriate action by the nurse?

A. Offer crackers and cheese.

B. Encourage sucking on eight hard candies.

C. Provide 8 oz of regular soda.

D. Give juice with table sugar.

4. A nurse is reinforcing dietary teaching to a client who has type 2 diabetes mellitus. Which of the following should the nurse include in the teaching? (Select all that apply.)

_____ A. Carbohydrates should comprise 55% of daily caloric intake.

_____ B. Use hydrogenated oils for cooking.

_____ C. Table sugar may be added to cereals.

_____ D. Drink an alcoholic beverage with meals.

_____ E. Protein foods can be substituted for carbohydrate foods.

5. A nurse is reviewing dietary guidelines to include in the plan of care for a client who has type 2 diabetes mellitus. Which of the following guidelines should the nurse include? (Select all that apply.)

_____ A. Weight management

_____ B. Lipid profile

_____ C. Cultural needs

_____ D. Sleep patterns

_____ E. Personal preferences

6. A nurse is reviewing the discharge plan for a client who has type 1 diabetes mellitus. How should interprofessional care be considered in the plan? Use the ATI Active Learning Template: Systems Disorder to complete this item to include the following:

A. Interprofessional Care: Describe the role of another member of the health care team.

B. Client Education: Describe three teaching points offered by this member.

APPLICATION EXERCISES KEY

1. A. **CORRECT:** Viral infections or certain genetic links may trigger an autoimmune response that causes type 1 diabetes mellitus.

    B. INCORRECT: Beta cells are damaged in type 1 diabetes mellitus.

    C. **CORRECT:** Type 1 diabetes mellitus usually occurs before age 30.

    D. INCORRECT: Type 1 diabetes mellitus is treated with insulin only.

    E. INCORRECT: Blood glucose is treated with insulin only. Diet and exercise may control blood glucose in type 2 diabetes mellitus.

    Ⓝ NCLEX® Connection: Physiological Adaptations, Illness Management

2. A. INCORRECT: Fruity breath odor is a manifestation of hyperglycemia.

    B. **CORRECT:** A client who has hypoglycemia may be diaphoretic.

    C. INCORRECT: Vomiting is not a manifestation of hyperglycemia or hypoglycemia.

    D. INCORRECT: Polyuria (excessive urination) is a manifestation of hyperglycemia.

    Ⓝ NCLEX® Connection: Reduction of Risk Potential, System Specific Assessments

3. A. INCORRECT: Crackers and cheese are offered when the blood glucose is in the expected reference range and the next meal is more than 1 hr away.

    B. **CORRECT:** Eight hard candies provides approximately 15 g of simple sugar to treat hypoglycemia.

    C. INCORRECT: The client should drink 4 oz of regular soda as a form of simple sugar to treat hypoglycemia.

    D. INCORRECT: The client should not take juice with table sugar, as the juice may slow the absorption of the simple sugar.

    Ⓝ NCLEX® Connection: Reduction of Risk Potential, System Specific Assessments

4. A. **CORRECT:** Carbohydrates should be 45% to 60% of total daily calorie intake.

    B. INCORRECT: Hydrogenated oils for cooking should be avoided because they contain trans fatty acids and cause hyperlipidemia.

    C. **CORRECT:** The client may use table sugar as long as adequate insulin or other agents are provided to cover the sugar intake.

    D. **CORRECT:** The client may drink an alcoholic beverage with meals or shortly after.

    E. INCORRECT: Carbohydrates can be exchanged but not with proteins.

    Ⓝ NCLEX® Connection: Physiological Adaptations, Illness Management

5. A. **CORRECT:** The nurse should include weight management in the plan of care if the client is overweight.

    B. **CORRECT:** The nurse should include the client's lipid profile to determine if a plan of care is needed for hyperlipidemia.

    C. **CORRECT:** The nurse should consider the client's cultural needs when developing a plan of care for management of type 2 diabetes mellitus.

    D. INCORRECT: A client's sleep pattern is not relevant in the plan of care for a client who has type 2 diabetes mellitus.

    E. **CORRECT:** The nurse should consider the client's personal preferences regarding food and activity when developing a plan of care for management of type 2 diabetes mellitus.

    Ⓝ NCLEX® Connection: Basic Care and Comfort, Nutrition and Oral Hydration

6. *Using the ATI Active Learning Template: Systems Disorder*

    A. Interprofessional Care
       • Dietician
          ○ Development of meal planning based on healthy food choices to meet the client's needs.

    B. Client Education
       • Review of exchange list: Incorporate proteins, carbohydrates, and fats within each group based on the client's needs.
       • Review of carbohydrate counting: Consider the total grams of carbohydrates in each food item and the quantity needed for each meal and snack.
       • Review information on food labels: Teach how to read food labels to identify amounts of carbohydrates contained in food.

    Ⓝ NCLEX® Connection: Physiological Adaptations, Illness Management

UNIT 3   ALTERATIONS IN NUTRITION

CHAPTER 16   Cancer and Immunosuppression Disorders

Overview

- Nurses should be knowledgeable of nutritional needs for clients who have cancer and immunosuppression disorders. Cancer can affect chewing, swallowing, satiety, digestion, nutrient absorption, use of glucose, and stool formation (dependent on type).

- Protein-calorie malnutrition and body wasting are the most common secondary diagnoses for clients who have cancer or immunosuppression disorders (human immunodeficiency virus [HIV]/acquired immunodeficiency syndrome [AIDS]). Nutritional deficits are a major cause of morbidity and mortality for these clients.

  - Adverse effects of treatments compromise the nutritional status of affected clients, and more than one-third of all cancer deaths are related to nutritional complications.

  - Immunosuppression disorders increase the body's nutrient demand, storage, and accessibility. They also cause loss of lean body tissue.

- The goals of nutritional therapy are to minimize the nutritional complications of disease, improve nutritional status, prevent muscle wasting, maintain weight, promote healing, reduce adverse effects, decrease morbidity and mortality, and enhance quality of life and the overall effectiveness of treatment therapies.

- Nutritional plans are individualized for client needs.

Assessment/Data Collection

- Subjective

  - History of current illness and presence of other medical diagnoses

  - Client's nutritional habits, food preferences, and restrictions

  - Food allergies

- Objective

  - Laboratory testing: albumin, ferritin, serum transferrin

  - Height, weight, body mass index (BMI), weight trends

Nutritional Guidelines and Nursing Interventions

- Nursing interventions for clients who are prescribed immunosuppression therapy or are immunocompromised

  - Instruct the client to avoid food sources of bacteria (raw fruits and vegetables, undercooked meat, poultry, or eggs). Wash, peel, and cook fruits and vegetables. Cook all foods thoroughly.

  - Monitor the effectiveness of nutrition (client weight, BMI, laboratory findings).

- ○ Teach the client to make appropriate food choices based on nutrition recommendations.
- ○ Assist the client to set realistic goals for nutrition and food consumption.
- ○ Instruct the client managing adverse effects of treatment.
- Cancer
  - ○ Excess body fat stimulates the production of estrogen and progesterone, which may intensify the growth of various cell types and may contribute to breast, gallbladder, colon, prostate, uterine, and kidney cancers.
  - ○ Preventative Nutrition
    - Consume adequate dietary fiber (14 grams per 1,000 kcal daily requirement) to lessen the risk of colon cancer.
    - Eliminate tobacco to reduce the risk of lung cancer.
    - Eat at least five servings of fruits and vegetables daily (linked to a lowered incidence of many types of cancer).
    - Consume whole grains rather than processed or refined grains and sugars. Gluten-free grains reduce the risk in some clients who have gastrointestinal disease.
    - Avoid meat prepared by smoking, pickling, charcoal grilling, and use of nitrate-containing chemicals (may be carcinogenic).
    - Consume polyunsaturated and monounsaturated fats (found in fish and olive oil) presumed to be beneficial in lowering the risk of many types of cancer.
    - Limit alcohol consumption (associated with many types of cancers).
    - A calcium-rich diet is associated with a lower incidence of colon cancer as it binds free fatty acids and bile salts in the lower gastrointestinal tract.
  - ○ Therapeutic Nutrition
    - Cancer may cause anorexia, increased metabolism, and negative nitrogen balance.
    - Systemic effects result in poor food intake, increased nutrient and energy needs, and catabolism of body tissues.

    - Creating an individualized plan for the client who has cancer is based on the following:
      - □ Increased caloric needs ranging from 25 to 35 cal/kg (dependent on metabolism, activity level, disease state, and ability to absorb nutrients).
      - □ Protein needs are increased to 1.0 to 2.5 g/kg.
      - □ Vitamin and mineral supplementation is based upon the client's needs.
    - Nursing Actions
      - □ Encourage clients to eat more on days when feeling better (on "good" days).
      - □ Encourage nutritional supplements that are high in protein and/or calories as between-meal snacks. When necessary, use as a meal replacement.
      - □ Increase protein and caloric content of foods by:
        - ‣ Substituting whole milk for water in recipes.
        - ‣ Adding milk, cheese, yogurt, or ice cream to dishes.
        - ‣ Using peanut butter as a spread for fruits.
        - ‣ Using yogurt as a topping for fruit.
        - ‣ Dipping meats in milk and bread crumbs before cooking.

▫ Treat complications associated with nutritional management

COMPLICATIONS	NUTRITIONAL MANAGEMENT INTERVENTIONS
Early satiety	› Eat small amounts of high-protein foods loaded with calories and nutrients.
Anorexia	› Eat small amounts of high-protein foods loaded with calories and nutrients. › Try to consume food in the morning when appetite is best. › Avoid food odors. › Do not fill up on low-calorie foods (broth, high-roughage foods containing water).
Mouth ulcers and stomatitis	› Use a soft toothbrush to clean teeth after eating and at bedtime. › Avoid mouth washes that contain alcohol. › Omit acidic, spicy, dry, or coarse foods. › Include cold or room temperature foods in the diet. › Cut food into small bites. › Try using straws. › Be sure dentures fit well.
Fatigue	› Eat a large, calorie-dense breakfast when energy level is the highest. › Conserve energy by eating foods that are easy to prepare. › Use a meal delivery service.
Food aversions	› Avoid eating foods that are well-tolerated and liked prior to treatments (chemotherapy, radiation).
Taste alterations and thick saliva	› Try adding foods that are tart (citrus juices). › Include cold or room temperature foods in the diet. › Try using sauces for added flavor. › Use plastic utensils for eating. › Suck on mints, candy, or chew gum to remove bad taste in mouth.
Gastrointestinal problems (nausea, vomiting, diarrhea)	› Nausea, vomiting » Eat cold or room temperature foods. » Try high-carbohydrate, low-fat foods. » Avoid fried foods. » Do not eat prior to chemotherapy or radiation. » Take prescribed antiemetic medication at the direction of the provider. › Diarrhea » Ensure adequate intake of liquids throughout the day to replace losses. » Avoid foods that may exacerbate diarrhea (foods high in roughage). » Consume foods high in pectin to increase the bulk of the stool and to lengthen transition time in the colon.

■ Teach client who has dysphagia how to promote swallowing: inhale, swallow, and then exhale and tilt the head.

- HIV/AIDS
  - Therapeutic Nutrition
    - The body's response to the inflammatory and immune processes associated with HIV increases nutrient requirements. Malnutrition is common and is one cause of death due to AIDS.
    - HIV infection, secondary infection, malignancies, and medication therapies can cause manifestations and adverse effects that impair intake and alter metabolism.
    - Creating an individualized plan for the client who has HIV/AIDS is based on the following:
      - □ Increased caloric needs, ranging from 35 to 55 cal/kg.
      - □ A high-protein diet is recommended with amounts varying from 1.2 to 2.0 g/kg.
      - □ The intake of a multivitamin that meets 100% of the recommended daily servings is sufficient, unless a specific deficiency is identified.
    - Decreased nutrient intake occurs because of physical manifestations (anorexia, nausea, vomiting, diarrhea). Psychological manifestations can include depression and dementia.
    - Nutritional warning findings in clients who have HIV/AIDS include rapid weight loss, gastrointestinal problems, inadequate intake, increased nutrient needs, food aversions, fad diets, and supplements.
    - If the client who has AIDS is unable to consume sufficient nutrients, calories, and fluid, enteral feedings may be needed.
    - Encourage the client to consume small, frequent meals that are composed of high-protein, high-calorie, and nutrient-dense foods.
    - Poor nutritional status leads to wasting and fever, further increasing susceptibility to secondary infections.
    - HIV associated wasting is characterized by unintended weight loss of 10% and at least one concurrent problem (diarrhea, chronic weakness, or fever) for at least 30 days.
    - Diarrhea and malabsorption are prominent clinical problems in clients who have AIDS.
    - Liberal fluid intake is extremely important to prevent dehydration.

APPLICATION EXERCISES

1. A nurse is teaching a client who has cancer about appropriate food choices. The nurse determines that the client understands the information when she chooses which of the following snacks? (Select all that apply.)

_____ A. Peanut butter sandwich on whole wheat bread with 2% milk

_____ B. Popcorn with soda

_____ C. Yogurt topped with granola and a banana

_____ D. Meat lasagna with buttered garlic bread

_____ E. Plain baked potato

2. A nurse is providing a community program on nutritional guidelines for cancer prevention. Which of the following should be included in the presentation? (Select all that apply.)

_____ A. Eating gluten-free grains may prevent cancer in clients who have gastrointestinal disorders.

_____ B. Adding dietary fiber lowers the risk of cancer.

_____ C. Charcoal grilling of meats is effective in preventing cancer.

_____ D. Using saturated cooking oil lowers the risk of cancer.

_____ E. Consuming low-calcium foods is associated with colon cancer.

3. A nurse in the oncology clinic is caring for a client who is undergoing treatment for cancer and reports difficulty eating due to inability to taste food. Which of the following is an appropriate intervention by the nurse?

A. Tell the client to avoid citrus juices.

B. Recommend that the client use plastic utensils when eating.

C. Discuss eating mostly heated or warmed foods.

D. Review adding foods high in pectin to the diet.

4. A nurse is teaching a client who is undergoing cancer treatment about interventions to manage stomatitis. Which of the following statements by the client indicates understanding of the teaching?

A. "I will try chewing larger pieces of food."

B. "I will avoid toasting my bread."

C. "I will consume more food in the morning."

D. "I will add more citrus foods to my diet."

5. A nurse is admitting a client who has suspected HIV-associated muscle wasting. Which of the following clinical manifestations supports this diagnosis?

    A. BMI of 26

    B. Fecal impaction

    C. Report of fever for 30 days

    D. Report of high alcohol consumption

6. A nurse in an oncology clinic is reviewing dietary management with a group of clients who have cancer and are undergoing treatment. What should be included in this discussion? Use the ATI Active Learning Template: Systems Disorder to complete this item to include the following:

    A. Client Education:
- Describe three effects of cancer on nutrition.
- Describe three nutrition needs.
- Describe three activities that promote improved nutrition.

APPLICATION EXERCISES KEY

1. A. **CORRECT:** These food choices reflect increased protein and calories for the client who has cancer.

    B. INCORRECT: These food choices do not provide needed protein for the client who has cancer.

    C. **CORRECT:** These food choices reflect increased protein and calories for the client who has cancer.

    D. **CORRECT:** These food choices reflect increased protein and calories for the client who has cancer.

    E. INCORRECT: This food choice contains carbohydrates, which provides calories, but is not a protein source, which is needed by the client who has cancer.

    Ⓝ NCLEX® Connection: Basic Care and Comfort, Nutrition and Oral Hydration

2. A. **CORRECT:** Consuming gluten-free grains reduces the risk of cancer in clients who have gastrointestinal disorders.

    B. **CORRECT:** Dietary fiber lessens the risk of colon cancer.

    C. INCORRECT: Charcoal grilling, smoking, and pickling may be carcinogenic.

    D. INCORRECT: The use of polyunsaturated and monounsaturated fats is beneficial in lowering the risk of many types of cancer.

    E. INCORRECT: A calcium-rich diet is associated with a lower incidence of colon cancer because it binds with free fatty acids and bile salts.

    Ⓝ NCLEX® Connection: Health Promotion and Maintenance, Health Promotion/Disease Prevention

3. A. INCORRECT: The client undergoing cancer treatment who has altered taste should add tart foods to the diet to promote improved taste sensation.

    B. **CORRECT:** The use of plastic utensils when eating may enhance taste sensations for the client undergoing cancer treatment.

    C. INCORRECT: The client undergoing cancer treatment who has altered taste may find that eating cold or room-temperature foods improves taste sensation.

    D. INCORRECT: The client undergoing cancer treatment and experiencing diarrhea should add pectin-rich foods to increase bulk of the stool and lengthen transition time in the colon.

    Ⓝ NCLEX® Connection: Basic Care and Comfort, Nutrition and Oral Hydration

4. A. INCORRECT: The client should be encouraged to cut food into small pieces to reduce irritation to mucous membranes.

    B. **CORRECT:** Dry, coarse foods such as toast can worsen the manifestations of stomatitis.

    C. INCORRECT: This intervention is appropriate for the client who has anorexia due to cancer treatment.

    D. INCORRECT: Acidic or spicy foods irritate the mucous membranes of the client who has stomatitis due to cancer treatment.

    (N) NCLEX® Connection: Basic Care and Comfort, Nutrition and Oral Hydration

5. A. INCORRECT: A BMI of 26 is within the expected reference range and is not a clinical finding in a client who has HIV-associated muscle wasting.

    B. INCORRECT: A client who has HIV-associated muscle wasting will report having diarrhea, not a fecal impaction, which is found in a client who has constipation.

    C. **CORRECT:** A client who has HIV-associated muscle wasting will report elevated temperature of over 30 days duration.

    D. INCORRECT: A client report of high alcohol consumption is not a clinical finding in HIV-associated muscle wasting.

    (N) NCLEX® Connection: Physiological Adaptations, Alterations in Body Systems

6. *Using the ATI Active Learning Template: Systems Disorder*

    A. Client Education:
    - Effects of cancer on nutrition: causes anorexia, increases metabolism, causes negative nitrogen balance.
    - Nutrition needs: increased calories (25 to 35 cal/kg), increased protein (1 to 2.5 g/kg), vitamin and mineral supplementation.
    - Activities
      ○ Eat more on days when feeling better.
      ○ Consume nutritional supplements that are high in protein and/or calories between meals and/or use as meal replacement.
      ○ Substitute whole milk for water in recipes.
      ○ Add milk, cheese, yogurt, or ice cream to foods when cooking.
      ○ Add peanut butter and yogurt as a spread/topping on fruits.
      ○ Coat meats in milk and bread crumbs before cooking.
      ○ Treat cancer-associated complications, such as early satiety, anorexia, mouth ulcers and stomatitis, fatigue, food aversions, altered taste, thick saliva, nausea, vomiting, and diarrhea.

    (N) NCLEX® Connection: Physiological Adaptations, Illness Management

REFERENCES

Dudek, S. G. (2010). *Nutrition essentials for nursing practice* (6th ed.). Philadelphia: Lippincott Williams & Wilkins.

Grodner, M., Roth, S. L., & Walkingshaw, B. C. (2012). *Nutrition Foundations and clinical applications of nutrition: A nursing approach* (5th ed.). St. Louis, MO: Mosby.

Hockenberry, M. J., & Winkelstein M. L. (2013). *Wong's essentials of pediatric nursing* (9th ed.). St. Louis, MO: Mosby.

Ignatavicius, D. D., & Workman, M. L. (2013). *Medical-surgical nursing* (7th ed.). St. Louis, MO: Saunders.

Lowdermilk, D. L., Perry, S. E., Cahsion, M. C., & Aldean, K. R. (2012). *Maternity & women's health care* (10th ed.). St. Louis, MO: Mosby.

Pillitteri, A. (2010). Maternal and child health nursing: *Care of the childbearing and childrearing family* (6th ed.). Philadelphia: Lippincott Williams & Wilkins.

Varcarolis, E. M., Carson, V. B., & Shoemaker, N. C. (2010). *Foundations of psychiatric mental health nursing: A clinical approach* (6th ed.). St. Louis, MO: Saunders.

CONTENT_____ REVIEW MODULE CHAPTER _____

TOPIC DESCRIPTOR_____

Related Content (e.g. delegation, levels of prevention, advance directives)	Underlying Principles	Nursing Interventions › Who? › When? › Why? › How?

Appendix

CONTENT _____ REVIEW MODULE CHAPTER _____

TOPIC DESCRIPTOR _____

DESCRIPTION OF PROCEDURE:

```
                    ┌─────────────────────────────┐
                    │        Procedure Name        │
                    └─────────────────────────────┘
```

Indications	Interpretation of Findings	Nursing Interventions (pre, intra, post)

```
              ┌─────────────────────────────┐
              │    Potential Complications    │
              └─────────────────────────────┘
```

Nursing Interventions	Client Education

Appendix

CONTENT _____ REVIEW MODULE CHAPTER _____

TOPIC DESCRIPTOR_____

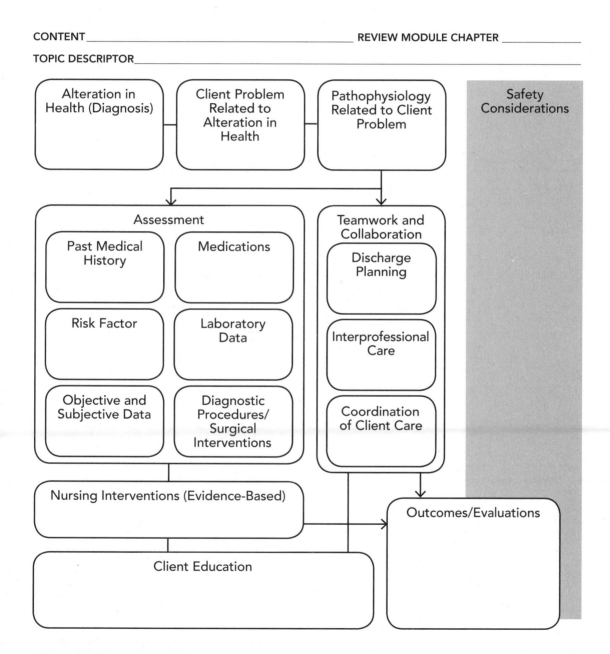

Appendix

CONTENT _____ REVIEW MODULE CHAPTER _____

TOPIC DESCRIPTOR_____

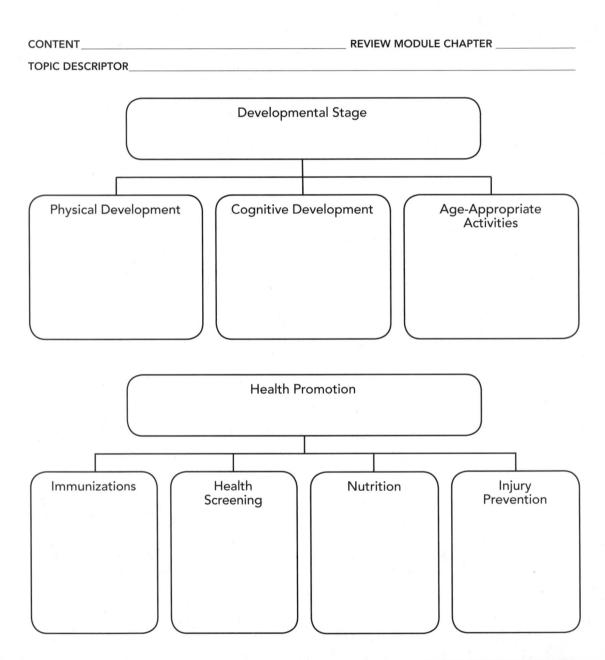

Developmental Stage

Physical Development

Cognitive Development

Age-Appropriate Activities

Health Promotion

Immunizations

Health Screening

Nutrition

Injury Prevention

Appendix

CONTENT _____ REVIEW MODULE CHAPTER _____

TOPIC DESCRIPTOR _____

MEDICATION _____

EXPECTED PHARMALOGICAL ACTION:

Therapeutic Uses

Adverse Effects

Nursing Interactions

Client Education

Client Education

Medication/Food Interactions

Nursing Administration

Evaluation of Medication Effectiveness

Appendix

CONTENT _____ REVIEW MODULE CHAPTER _____

TOPIC DESCRIPTOR_____

DESCRIPTION OF SKILL:

```
                        ┌─────────────────────────────┐
                        │        Procedure Name        │
                        └─────────────────────────────┘
```

Indications	Nursing Interventions (pre, intra, post)	Outcomes/Evaluations

```
                        ┌─────────────────────────────┐
                        │     Potential Complications   │
                        └─────────────────────────────┘
```

Nursing Interventions	Client Education

Appendix

CONTENT_____ REVIEW MODULE CHAPTER _____

TOPIC DESCRIPTOR_____

DESCRIPTION OF PROCEDURE:

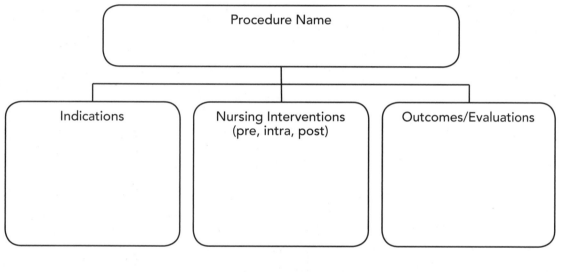

Procedure Name

Indications

Nursing Interventions
(pre, intra, post)

Outcomes/Evaluations

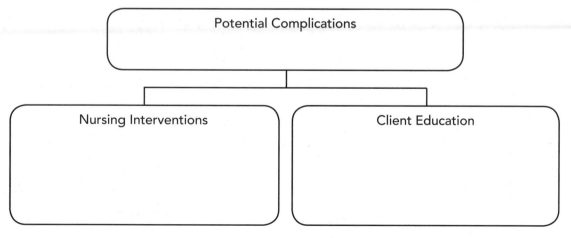

Potential Complications

Nursing Interventions

Client Education